NEW LIBRARY OF PSYCHOANALYSIS

General editor: Elizabeth Bott Spillius

Michael Balint

Object Relations Pure and Applied

Harold Stewart

with chapters by
Andrew Elder and Robert Gosling

For Barbara,
Brian and Rosalind

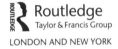

Routledge
Taylor & Francis Group

LONDON AND NEW YORK

First published 1996 by Routledge
27 Church Road, Hove, East Sussex BN3 2FA
711 Third Avenue, New York NY 10017

Routledge is an imprint of the Taylor & Francis Group, an informa business

Typeset in Times by LaserScript, Mitcham, Surrey

British Library Cataloguing in Publication Data
A catalogue record for this book is available from the British Library.

Library of Congress Cataloging-in-Publication Data are available

ISBN 13: 978–0–415–14466–7 (pbk)

Michael Balint

While Michael Balint's applied work is widely known, many of his theoretical contributions have been incorporated into everyday analysis without due recognition of their source. In this account of his thinking, Harold Stewart evaluates the extent of Balint's contribution to psychoanalysis and firmly re-establishes his place within the development of object relations theory.

The first part examines Balint's theories of human psychological development, defining such concepts as primary love, ocnophilia and philobatism, the basic fault and the three areas of the mind. The author places Balint's understanding of the analyst's influence and technique and of therapeutic regression in the context of his relationship with Sandor Ferenczi, his analyst and mentor. The second part looks at how the 'Balint group' has contributed to the assessment and understanding of emotional problems in various arenas, including general practice, marital work and psychosexual medicine. Balint was a charismatic teacher, and his work with general practitioners has become an established, world-wide institution. Features of this work, including the use of counter-transference and the affective response of the doctor, are vividly described here by Andrew Elder and Robert Gosling.

Michael Balint: Object Relations Pure and Applied brings alive Balint's teaching and practice and demonstrates the relevance of his theories to many of the problematic issues in current analytic practice.

Harold Stewart was training analyst and supervisor at the British Psycho-Analytical Society and author of *Psychic Experience and Problems of Technique*, also in this series.

THE NEW LIBRARY OF PSYCHOANALYSIS
General Editor Dana Birksted-Breen

The New Library of Psychoanalysis was launched in 1987 in association with the Institute of Psychoanalysis, London. It took over from the International Psychoanalytical Library, which published many of the early translations of the works of Freud and the writings of most of the leading British and Continental psychoanalysts.

The purpose of the New Library of Psychoanalysis is to facilitate a greater and more widespread appreciation of psychoanalysis and to provide a forum for increasing mutual understanding between psychoanalysts and those working in other disciplines such as the social sciences, medicine, philosophy, history, linguistics, literature and the arts. It aims to represent different trends both in British psychoanalysis and in psychoanalysis generally. The New Library of Psychoanalysis is well placed to make available to the English-speaking world psychoanalytic writings from other European countries and to increase the interchange of ideas between British and American psychoanalysts.

The Institute, together with the British Psychoanalytical Society, runs a low-fee psychoanalytic clinic, organizes lectures and scientific events concerned with psychoanalysis and publishes the *International Journal of Psychoanalysis*. It also runs the only UK training course in psychoanalysis that leads to membership of the International Psychoanalytical Association – the body which preserves internationally agreed standards of training, of professional entry, and of professional ethics and practice for psychoanalysis as initiated and developed by Sigmund Freud. Distinguished members of the Institute have included Michael Balint, Wilfred Bion, Ronald Fairbairn, Anna Freud, Ernest Jones, Melanie Klein, John Rickman and Donald Winnicott.

Previous General Editors include David Tuckett, Elizabeth Spillius and Susan Budd. Previous and current Members of the Advisory Board include Christopher Bollas, Ronald Britton, Donald Campbell, Stephen Grosz, John Keene, Eglé Laufer, Juliet Mitchell, Michael Parsons, Rosine Jozef Perelberg, David Taylor, Mary Target, Catalina Bronstein, Sara Flanders and Richard Rusbridger.

ALSO IN THIS SERIES

Contents

Preface

Michael Balint was one of the group of creative analysts who, working in the context of the British Psycho-Analytical Society, developed and advanced what is known as the British object relations school of psychoanalysis. He, together with Melanie Klein, Donald Winnicott, Ronald Fairbairn and Wilfred Bion, developed the theory that the subject's need to relate to objects is of central importance to the subject, which contrasts with instinct theory, in which the subject's need is for the reduction of instinctual tension. Each of these pioneers had their own views and theories on the nature and development of these needs from earliest infancy onwards, and in this book those of Balint as set out in his writings will be examined. Since theory and technique for conducting an analysis are intimately interlinked, his views on the nature and developments of technique will constitute an essential part of this study.

This book is not a biography, although it includes a brief biographical sketch of his life. It is essentially a study of his work in the twin fields of pure and applied psychoanalysis. In the latter, his work, with general practitioners in particular, was deservedly world-famous, and to mark this, three chapters are devoted to this topic. Two of the three are written by Dr Robert Gosling, psychoanalyst, former director of the Tavistock Clinic, and an early colleague of Balint, working with him in the development of his general practitioner groups. The other chapter is written by Dr Andrew Elder, general practitioner, member of the Balint Society, and a more contemporary member of the Balint groups.

I have written this book as a homage and tribute to Michael Balint, my analytic grandfather, the supervisor of my first training case, and above all, the person who set me firmly on the road to psychoanalysis. If there are any errors, omissions or misrepresentation of his views, the responsibility rests solely with me.

I would like to acknowledge the help and proddings of my editor, Elizabeth Spillius, and the assistance and efficiency of my secretary, Helen Abbott.

Harold Stewart

Biographical sketch

Michael Balint was born in Budapest on 3 December 1896. He came from a middle-class Jewish family, the family name being Bergsmann. His father was a general practitioner, practising in Josefstadt, the largely Jewish quarter of Budapest, and it was here that he spent his formative years. On growing up, he changed his name to the more Hungarian one of Balint and was also converted to the Unitarian faith. (I am indebted to André Haynal's book *The Technique at Issue* for many of these facts.) He had a younger sister, Emmi, who studied mathematics and was at school with two future analysts, Margaret Mahler and Alice Szekely-Kovacs, his future wife.

He enrolled as a medical student but soon afterwards was conscripted for military service at the outbreak of the First World War in 1914. He saw active service in Russia and Italy but was then severely wounded in the hand, giving it a rather claw-like deformity. The injury was thought to be either self-inflicted to escape military service or the result of foolhardiness in allowing his natural curiosity to get the better of him by trying to dismantle a hand-grenade. Whichever it was, he was discharged from the army and resumed his medical studies, qualifying as a doctor in 1918, with a special interest in biology and biochemistry. As a student he had read *The Interpretation of Dreams* and *The Psychopathology of Everyday Life* and was ambivalently critical of them, but in 1917 he was conquered for psycho-analysis by *Three Essays on Sexuality* and *Totem and Taboo*, with two topics, the development of sexual functioning and the development of human relations, remaining the focus of his future work. Shortly after qualifica-tion, he married Alice, and their relationship, living and working together, was extremely harmonious.

Following the end of the First World War in 1918, the Communist Republic of Bela Kun was established in Hungary and was actively sup-ported by the young progressives such as Balint. By 1919, the regime had been overthrown and Balint's future became uncertain, which resulted in his leaving Budapest for Berlin. Here he worked at the Berlin Psychoanalytic

1

Institute conducting psychoanalytic treatments, and also at the Berlin Charité Hospital treating psychosomatic cases. This made him one of the very first people treating psychosomatic disorders by psychoanalysis. In 1922 he went into analysis himself with Hans Sachs, but after two years he decided that Sachs was too didactic in his approach and terminated his analysis. (He once told me that he could always remember, with great dislike, Sachs' telephone number, since he would answer telephone calls during sessions, starting with the number.)

Accordingly, in 1924 he returned to Budapest and entered analysis with Sandor Ferenczi, as did Alice. This analysis also lasted two years, but this time it was terminated when Ferenczi went to New York for eight months. In this period, Balint felt himself to be an analyst, and this is evidenced by the fact that his publications changed from being on bacteriology and biochemistry to the subject of psychoanalysis. He then became a member of the Hungarian Psychoanalytical Society, helped in 1930 to establish the Psychoanalytic Out-Patient Clinic in Budapest, became vice-director of the Budapest Psychoanalytic Institute from 1931 to 1935, and from 1935 to 1939, its director.

In 1932, the Hungarian government came to resemble a racist, pro-Hitler state, and Balint gives a fascinating account of the working atmosphere created by this:

> in the thirties . . . the political situation in Hungary became tenser every day. It seemed most unlikely that any institution could offer me facilities for testing out my ideas so I decided to gather a few general practitioners in a kind of seminar for the study of psychotherapeutic possibilities in their practice. Although I had only vague ideas of what was needed by my colleagues – e.g. I started the seminar with a series of lectures, which I know now are quite useless – the interest remained alive and even a second group was formed. However, the political situation deteriorated further; we were ordered to notify the police of every one of our meetings with the result that a plain-clothes policeman attended each of them, taking copious notes of everything that was said. We could never find out what these notes contained or who read them. The only result we knew of was that on several occasions the detective, after the meeting, consulted one of us either about himself, his wife, or his children. This was quite amusing for us, but no proper discussions could develop under these circumstances and the group of doctors disintegrated eventually.
>
> (1970: 458)

Here we see the origins of the future 'Balint groups' used in a number of allied disciplines.

In 1938 at the time of the Austrian *Anschluss*, Freud and his family came to England, and soon afterwards, with the help of Ernest Jones and John Rickman, Michael, Alice and their son, John, arrived in Manchester, where they took up residence in 1939. Tragically, shortly afterwards in August 1939, Alice, aged 40 years, died suddenly of a ruptured aortic aneurysm, a looming danger of which both she and Michael had long been aware.

He continued to live in Manchester and obtained his British medical qualifications, enabling him to practise in Great Britain. This was followed by a postgraduate Master of Science degree in psychology with a thesis on 'Individual Differences in Early Infancy', a study of infants' feeding rhythms. He was appointed consultant psychiatrist to the Manchester Northern Royal Hospital, and director of two child guidance clinics, the North East Lancashire and the County Borough of Preston Child Guidance Clinics (1944, 1945). In 1945 he came to London and was director of Chislehurst Child Guidance Clinic from 1945 to 1947.

Just before his move to London in 1945, he married his second wife, Edna Oakeshott. However, they separated in 1947 and divorced in 1952. In 1953, he married his third wife, Enid Eichholz, née Albu, with whom he had a similarly harmonious marriage to that with Alice.

In 1945, he was notified of the tragic circumstances of his parents' death. They had committed suicide by lethal injections of morphine when they were about to be arrested by the Hungarian Nazis, rather than face the certain fate of the gas chambers. In a letter of 15 January 1945 to Alice's sister, Olga Dormandi, he wrote:

> It is true that I had neglected my father for a long time. We never got along too well. We were never really on good terms. But I had inherited my intelligence, my logical mind, my capacity for work from him. I loved my mother very much. She was so in touch with life; things never worked out well for her and still she never gave up hope.
>
> (Haynal 1988: 112)

In 1947, he became a British subject and in 1948 he joined the staff of the Tavistock Clinic, and it was from there that most of his world-famous work in the field of applied psychoanalysis took shape as he continued the work that had its origins in pre-war Budapest. The Clinic, together with the Tavistock Institute of Human Relations, was re-organizing after the war and included a number of analysts and candidates on its staff. Their main concern, apart from offering a psychotherapeutic service for patients in the National Health Service, was the study of interpersonal relationships, their origins and development in the context of the family, and their nature within groups and organizations of different kinds.

In 1948, a group of social workers in the Family Welfare Association in collaboration with the staff of the Tavistock Institute created the Family Discussion Bureau to provide facilities for those who sought help with their own marital problems and for professional workers to study the development of techniques for dealing with these problems. The leader of the social workers' group was Mrs Enid Eichholz, the future Mrs Michael Balint, and the co-founder of the Bureau was Michael Balint. Together they developed the 'case discussion seminar', which became the vehicle for the basic psychological training in this and other disciplines. The Bureau grew and developed and eventually in 1968 became the present Institute of Marital Studies.

In 1950, Balint instituted 'Research cum Training' seminars for general practitioners who wanted to get a better understanding of the emotional problems that they met in the course of everyday practice. This, of course, had its origins too in the seminars for general practitioners in Budapest. This work in many ways has changed the face of general practice not only in this country but throughout the world. In 1952, he started similar seminars for the treatment of psychosexual disorders with the Family Planning Association, later to become the Institute of Psychosexual Studies. In 1955, he set up a brief psychotherapy workshop with analysts from the Tavistock Clinic and the Cassel Hospital to develop brief focal psychotherapy.

In 1961, he had to retire from the Tavistock Clinic since he had reached the retiring age of 65 years, but he immediately joined the staff of University College Hospital, where he started his case discussion groups, for medical students. The seminars with general practitioners and medical students, the 'Balint groups', continued until his death. Prior to this, in 1969, the general practitioners of the Balint groups founded the Balint Society for the discussion and advancement of this work.

Every year from 1958 onwards, he and Enid went to Cincinnati, Ohio, he as visiting professor and she as associate professor, where they continued their work and teaching, particularly with Paul Ornstein. Balint had also been President of the Medical Section of the British Psychological Society. Within the British Psycho-Analytical Society, where he was a training analyst of the Independent (Middle) Group, he was elected Scientific Secretary for 1951–53, and later President, from 1968 until his death on 31 December 1970. During his presidency, he initiated the popular biennial meetings, the English-Speaking Conferences of the European Psychoanalytical Federation. He died, while in office, of a severe coronary infarction from which he appeared to have recovered, but shortly after leaving hospital, collapsed and died. He was 74 years of age. Since then, his work has been carried on by Enid until her recent death, on 30 July 1994.

Michael Balint was kind, generous, understanding and averse to authoritarianism. He could also be provocative, high-handed, scornful and

4

authoritarian. He could be loved or hated but it was difficult to be indifferent to him. He greatly valued independence of thought, together with strong argument, and, to use his own terminology, he had much of the 'philobat' in him. Such people are essential if psychoanalysis is to continue to develop.

Introduction

Michael Balint, one of the most searching and innovative members of the second generation of psychoanalysts, was a product of the Budapest School of Psychoanalysis and the analysand of its founder, Sandor Ferenczi. I first met him at the Tavistock Clinic in the 1950s, then at its home in Beaumont Street, W1, in the Harley Street area, when I went to see him for advice on psychotherapy training. He was then a solid middle-aged man of medium height with a marked Hungarian accent and a direct and forthright manner. When he was later the supervisor of my first psycho-analytical training case, I came to value this directness, together with his ability to admit error; yet others occasionally found him rather bullying, particularly in seminars, although this was a trait I never experienced with him. However, we all acknowledged his capacity to challenge and question everything, never to take things for granted, in order to help people to think for themselves, and in this respect he resembled both Ferenczi and Freud. Ferenczi, the master in his time of psychoanalytic technique and experimentation, the fearless theoretician, was the model other than Freud on which Balint based himself as an analyst. Throughout his life, he acknowledged his unresolved positive transference and indebtedness to him. In a way following his mentors, the main directions of his researches were in the development of human relationships and of individual sexual functioning. Unlike them, his approach was less speculative, being more derived through his clinical observations of the analytic situation and the influence of psychoanalytic technique on both patient and analyst.

In the three fields, object relationships, sexuality and psychoanalytic technique, his views and concepts developed over a period of some forty years, and the aim of the first part of this book is to give an account of these developments as recorded in his published works. He was not a tidy thinker. His ideas were developed piecemeal over the years and he was not very much concerned if they were incomplete and not closely integrated with any main corpus of theory. The nearest he came to such an integration was in his final book, *The Basic Fault* (1968). The first part of this present book will be devoted to his work in the psychoanalytic field proper and the second to his almost equally important work in the field of applied psychoanalysis. This introduction will mainly be devoted to giving a brief outline of his theories and ideas in clinical psychoanalysis, which will then be examined in greater detail in the following chapters.

Some of his most important contributions to theory and technique lie within the concept of *regression*, particularly in its use as a therapeutic agent in psychoanalysis. Balint did not introduce the concept of regression, of going backwards in the mind to earlier and more primitive modes of functioning. This originated with Freud, who introduced the concepts of topographical, temporal and formal regression, and it was later developed by Ferenczi for its potential as a therapeutic agent. Freud, as a consequence of the use made of regressive techniques by Ferenczi, came to disagree with it, and Melanie Klein, in view of her belief that regression is solely a defence and not something valuable in its own right, concurred with Freud. It was, however, Balint, together with Donald Winnicott, who as members of the British Psycho-Analytical Society did most to develop and refine theories and techniques on this issue.

The topic of regression, the return to the more primitive, is intimately associated with the theories of the development of object relationships from infancy, of the relationship of the self with the environment and particularly the primary objects in that environment. Balint's first mention of regression was in his second psychoanalytical paper, 'Psychosexual Parallels to the Fundamental Law of Biogenetics' (1930), which developed the concept, not in its clinical sense but in a biological context, an appropriate one befitting an analyst whose first discipline before medicine and psychoanalysis was biology. Interestingly, though, this paper also introduced the first of his original concepts, that of the *new beginning*. This refers to the opportunity in the analysis for the patient to learn anew fresh ways of loving, with the dropping of pathological compulsive patterns that had previously been the only ones available. This concept is somewhat similar to Freud's concept of working-through and Klein's views on mourning and reparation, although this latter concept is used only once by Balint. In this biological paper, however, new beginning was only used in the biological sense of the progressive development of new structures and functions from older ones.

His thinking on these two related concepts, regression and new begin-ning, was developed in his next paper, 'Character Analysis and New Beginning' (1932), where he describes his clinical experiences of work with regressed patients, and significantly, in the light of his further thinking on regression, describes some of the difficulties and problems that are encountered in the clinical work with these patients. Here is the seed from which his major contribution in the field evolved, his distinction between two types of regression, *benign regression* and *malignant regression*, which was first described in his last book, *The Basic Fault* (1968). This distinction between the two types is very important clinically because, as the terms 'benign' and 'malignant' indicate, one is helpful therapeutically whereas the other is potentially dangerous and destructive to the continuity of the analysis (and, of course, any other form of psychotherapy).

Between the 1932 paper and *The Basic Fault*, there are occasional references to regression, but the other main discussion on the topic is in his third book, *Thrills and Regressions* (1959a). Balint looks at regression from its theoretical aspect concerning its relationship to early forms of object relationships with their influence on the development of the individual psyche. He had long had his own views on these early states of development. He did not hold with Freud's concept of primary narcissism, and strongly argued that *narcissism is always a secondary phenomenon*, that narcissism always means secondary narcissism. This view was first put forward in his paper 'Critical Notes on the Theory of the Pregenital Organizations of the Libido' (1935b), developed further in 'Early Developmental States of the Ego: Primary Object-love' (1937b), and most fully in *The Basic Fault* (1968). He believed, as had Ferenczi, that the object relationship of the infant to its mother is primary, is a basic biological and psychological given, and is present in the very earliest, deepest and most primitive layers of the mind. Winnicott continued to accept Freud's view, whereas Klein soon followed Balint in his rejection of primary narcissism. At first, in 'Critical Notes' (1935), following Ferenczi, he describes this primary stage as *passive object-love*, the aim of which for the infant is being loved unconditionally by the mother, with the biological basis being the instinctual interdependence of mother and child. However, in the paper on 'Primary Object-love' (1937b), in view of his recognition that this state is not simply passive but contains many active features, he changed it from 'passive' to '*primary object-love*'. This primitive state of primary love is described in *Thrills and Regressions* (1959a) as a state of *harmonious mix-up* of subject and object. Under the influence of the inevitable frustrations by, and separations from, the object, the other, this harmonious world is destroyed and discrete, firm objects emerge. He postulated that in response to these traumatic events, the infant may develop in the direction of what he termed *ocnophilia* or of *philobatism* in its object relationships. By the term 'ocnophilia' he meant that objects are experienced as being friendly and safe whereas the spaces between objects are experienced as being threatening and hostile; in philobatism, the objects are experienced as threatening and hostile, with the spaces between them being experienced as safe and friendly. These configurations are the basis of the two character types, the *ocnophiles* and the *philobats*, whose characteristics and pathology are extensively delineated in *Thrills and Regressions* (1959a). However, by his choice of these awkward-sounding and difficult words, Balint did himself a disservice, since they are difficult to remember. This meant that the actual concepts concerning objects and the space between them also fail to be remembered and used in psychoanalysts' thinking.

In a later development, he adds, in *The Basic Fault* (1968), an intermediate stage between primary object-love and ocnophilia–philobatism, and this is the stage of the *basic fault*. It was first introduced as a concept in his paper, 'The Doctor, His Patient and the Illness' (1955b), which was also used as the title of his book on his work with general practitioners, but was extensively developed in his book of that name. The basic fault is conceptualized as a structural deficiency in the mind, a fault in the geological and not the moral sense, originating from considerable early discrepancies between the bio-psychological needs of the infant and the material and psychological care and affection of the primary objects. It is from the intensity of these early discrepant experiences and their associated phantasies that the states of ocnophilia–philobatism arise, and it is to these experiences and phantasies, together with their later derivatives, that regressions occur. It is also to the new beginning from these states that emotional growth and development can resume again. Freud and Klein in their theories of development do not use the ideas of a fault or a deficit in relation to the primary object. Winnicott (1952) uses the concept in his theory of impingement and the development of a false-self organization, and interestingly, Bion (1962) in his 'Theory of Thinking' also formulates a deficiency of the containing object in the provision of alpha-functioning for the infant.

To return to his early paper on 'Critical Notes on the Theory of Pregenital Organizations of the Libido' (1935b), he suggests that the aim of all erotic striving is to achieve the harmonious state with the object, the feeling of unity with it, as is found in primary object-love. When this state is inevitably disturbed, he suggests that there are two non-pathological secondary routes that could lead back to that ego-state. The first is via narcissism: if I am not loved, I have to love myself; and the second is via active object-love: I have to love and gratify my partner in order to be loved and gratified by him in return. These constitute the normal paths of the development of object relations as compared with the early pathological states of ocnophilia and philobatism. All of these states have been concerned with vicissitudes of loving and of the libido, and it is not until his paper 'On Love and Hate' (1951) that he puts forward a *theory of hate*. In his opinion, hate is always of a reactive secondary nature and not one of the basic primary drives of the individual, and his theory was that hate is the last remnant, the denial of, and the defence against, the primary object-love. In proposing the secondary nature of hate and destructivity,

9

Balint differs from Freud, Klein and Winnicott. Fairbairn, however, concurs with Balint in this view.

In his theories of primitive object relationships, Balint concentrated largely on the understanding of the two-person relationship, commencing with the infant–mother dyad of primary love and leading on to the basic fault and the two character types, ocnophilia and philobatism. In *The Basic Fault*, he introduced a new theory of the mind concerning the topic of object relations called the *three areas of the mind*. These three areas are conceptualized in terms of one-person, two-person and three-person relationships. The one-person relationship is described as the *area of creation*, the two-person relationship as the *area of the basic fault*, and the three-person relationship as the *area of the Oedipus conflict*. The area of creation relates to artistic and scientific activity, to insight and understanding, and to the early phases of becoming physically or mentally ill and of spontaneous recovery from them. The area relates to *pre-objects*, which are neither organized nor whole objects, until they are externalized as creations. The area of the basic fault has as its dynamic force the structural deficiency in the mind; the area of the Oedipus conflict is characterized by triangular relationships and the dynamic force operating at this level is mental conflict. Each of these areas is described in terms of its own observed characteristics and qualities on which this differentiation of these three areas has been based.

In addition to his contributions to psychoanalytical theory, Balint made several contributions to technique. He was one of the earliest writers to discuss the phenomenon of *counter-transference*. In 'On Transference of Emotions' (1933d), counter-transference is equated by him with the analyst's own transference to the patient. Six years later, in 'On Transference and Counter-transference' (1939a), it included everything in the analytical situation that reveals the personality of the analyst. In 'Changing Thera-peutical Aims and Techniques in Psychoanalysis' (1949), he now takes counter-transference to mean the totality of the analyst's analytical behaviour and professional attitude towards the patient. This last paper particularly emphasizes Balint's belief that one of the most important fields of investigation in psychoanalysis is the *analyst's behaviour in the analytical situation, their contribution to the creating and maintaining of this situation*. By this he includes three interrelated aspects of the situation. First, there is the analytic language of the particular analyst, the set of technical terms, concepts, models and frames of reference that he uses in order to construct his interpretations. Second, he includes the analyst's behaviour in terms of the emotional tension aroused, and the consideration of the *necessary frustrations and satisfactions* that are needed to maintain this tension at an optimal level. Third, he includes the *creating of a proper atmosphere* to enable patients to express and reveal themselves optimally.

These last two features, the consideration of necessary frustrations and satisfactions and the creating of a proper atmosphere, are considerably developed in *The Basic Fault*, where the issues involved in therapeutic regression are described, since it is in states of regression that these two features assume particular importance. The main issue is whether regression and regressive behaviour in analysis is conceptualized as a defence against the immediacy, the here-and-now, of the transference situation, or whether it is regarded not simply as a defence but also as an important communication to the analyst of a state of mind concerning deeply regressed traumatic experiences of the patient, whether real or phantasied, or some derivative of it. If it is regarded as a defence, then interpretation of its defensive nature in the transference will be the analyst's technical procedure. If, however, it is regarded as a regression to explore the significance of where it may lead, then only after the patient emerges from the regressed state will the necessary interpretative work take place. This is Balint's position, and he believes that the attitude and behaviour of the analyst in this role is not simply that of providing interpretations but of creating the appropriate atmosphere for regression to be allowed to occur. He describes this attitude as the *unobtrusive analyst*, with the analyst being pliant and flexible in their technique and at the same time being indestructible in their professional stance as an analyst. This view of the unobtrusive analyst and the proper atmosphere created is clearly related to his concept of primary love and the harmonious object relationship and feeling of oneness that accompanies it.

His last contribution to psychoanalytic theory is a new *theory of trauma*. His paper, 'Trauma and Object Relationship' (1969), describes trauma as having a triphasic structure and is based on Ferenczi's views of traumatogenesis in childhood. The first phase is a trusting loving one between child and adult, which is followed by the second phase in which the adult does something frightening, exciting or painful to the child resulting in severe overstimulation of the child. The trauma is then caused particularly by the third phase in which the adult reacts with indifference towards the child's appeals or protests.

To turn to the field of applied psychoanalysis, Balint's major contribution was in the field of general medical practice. In the early 1950s, he established discussion groups for interested general practitioners to examine problems that had arisen in the course of their work with patients in their practices and the ways that these problems might be handled by the doctor. Balint was a charismatic figure for the members of his groups, which was no doubt due to his qualities of directness and enquiry, to his ability to empathize with their difficulties and problems in the work situation, and to his ability to formulate concepts which captured their experience of general practice. In some measure, this was due to the fact that his father had been a general practitioner in Budapest, which must have given Michael early experience of the work, and also to the fact that Ferenczi had interested himself in the work of Hungarian general practitioners. These discussion groups were eventually called *Balint groups* and the doctors involved instituted a *Balint Society* in 1969 to discuss and continue his work. His major account of this work is his internationally famous book, *The Doctor, His Patient and the Illness* (1957a), in which he introduced the ideas of the *doctor as the important drug* whose dosage and frequency needed determining, the importance of the *initial complaining* of the patient, and the *apostolic function of the doctor*, meaning his attitudes and responses to the patient's complaints and his expectations of the patient. His basic premise was that any emotion felt by the doctor in his immediate relationship with the patient needed to be regarded as a symptom of the illness. The relationship of these concepts to those used in the analytic context are closely interrelated, particularly in his original use of the emotional response in the doctor's counter-transference for patients in general practice.

In addition to general practitioners, he used this form of discussion group in other contexts, particularly with psychoanalytic colleagues to study the use and application of brief focal psychotherapy techniques in the National Health Service, and with doctors and nurses working in the Family Planning Association, which became the Institute of Psycho-sexual Medicine.

Much of his work in these applied fields and also in his later psycho-analytic work was done in partnership with his wife, Enid, who was also a considerable theorist in her own right, and she had continued his applied work since his death in 1970 with the general practitioners in particular. Their joint books, some including other colleagues as co-authors, are *Psychotherapeutic Techniques in Medicine* (1961), *A Study of Doctors* (1966a), and *Focal Psychotherapy* (1972), and these books continue the themes of the work with general practitioners and the brief methods of psychotherapy.

This introduction will now be followed by a more detailed examination of his work.

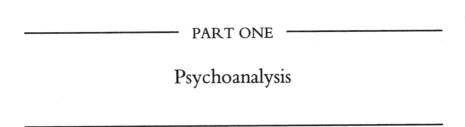

PART ONE

Psychoanalysis

1

Primary Love and Psychoanalytic Technique (1952)

This book contains the papers that represent Balint's contributions to the theory and practice of psychoanalysis from the years 1930 to 1952 and I shall consider those that seem most relevant to the general thrust of his thinking. In the Preface, he gives a brief overall view of his work:

> After having ambivalently criticized The Interpretation of Dreams and The Psychopathology of Everyday Life, I was at the age of 21 decisively and definitely conquered for psychoanalysis by the Three Contributions and Totem and Taboo. In some form or other, these two directions of research – the development of the individual sexual function and the development of human relationships – have remained in the focus of my interest ever since. Coming from medicine, and strongly biased by my predilection for the exact sciences, my approach to these two problems was mainly, though not exclusively, through clinical observation; this meant studying the processes as they develop and change under the impact of the analytical situation in the patient, that is, studying the psychoanalyst's technique and the patient's responses to it. This volume collects my papers written during the years 1930–1952 on these three intimately interlinked topics – human sexuality, object-relations, and psychoanalytic technique.
>
> (1952a: 5)

It would be true to say that all of his subsequent publications continued the task of researching and exploring these three topics.

His very first psychoanalytic paper, 'Perversion or a Hysterical Symptom?', was written in 1925 and is not included in this book but is published in his second volume, *Problems of Human Pleasure and Behaviour* (1956). It concerns the topic of homosexuality, and it gives a brief clinical account of whether a patient's symptoms should be considered a perversion or hysterical in nature. It already reveals his enquiring and questioning mind, particularly in the highlighting of the deficiencies and limitations of the current knowledge of psychoanalysis at the time of writing. Like Freud, he was always aware of the present limits of psychoanalytic understanding and of the need for continual probing and research to extend the limits.

'Psychosexual Parallels to the Fundamental Law of Biogenetics', published in 1930, was his next paper and is the first in the book. He discusses the development of psychosexuality in terms of the biological development of the species. The relationship between psychosexual development and the biological development of different forms of animal life from the most simple and primitive had particularly interested Ferenczi, who developed these ideas in his book *Thalassa: A Theory of Genitality* (1938), an original and unique contribution to psychoanalytic thinking and speculation. Balint, who often proclaims his positive transference feelings to his analyst and mentor, is clearly impressed by Ferenczi's thinking in the writing of his own paper. The fundamental law of biogenetics as formulated by Ernst Haeckel postulates that the development of the individual from the initial fertilization of the egg repeats the evolutionary development of the race, phylogenesis, or to use Balint's adaptation of this: 'The fertilized human egg knows all about phylogenesis; it recapitulates it in its own development' (1952a: 11). This refers only to the body, but Balint develops the theme to include the development of the mind, which is also recapitulating the development of the species, and he uses the development of psychosexual phases, as described by Freud and Abraham, to further his ideas. They are developed in some biological detail, as befits a psychoanalyst whose first professional training was as a biologist.

An interesting feature of this paper is that it introduces two concepts, both in biological terms, that he develops later in terms of psychology. These are *regression* and *new beginning*. He points out that in the process of reproduction, the cells after union become more primitive in nature, and suggests 'that the organism regresses to an earlier stage of evolution, returning to long-abandoned life-forms, in order to begin its existence anew from there' (1952a: 37). He then suggests that 'This *new beginning* plays a very important part in the living world. The development of each fertilized egg represents a new beginning' (1952a: 37). This concept of regression to something earlier and more primitive, together with the stage of being followed by a new beginning of further development, is to become of major importance in his contributions to theory and technique. In fact, his next paper, in 1932, is entitled 'Character Analysis and New Beginning' and deals precisely with these issues.

He opens with the observation that patients are no longer satisfied with the removal of symptoms and wish to continue their treatment after this has occurred. He believes that they 'wish, often unconsciously, to be able to love free from anxiety and lose their fear of complete surrender' (1952a: 159). Furthermore, some patients represent a new type of patient whose suffering is often not of symptoms but of getting little pleasure from anything in life. Such patients are afraid of excitation, even of the gratifying pleasure itself. Analytic work always leads back to childhood situations, either with adults evoking sexual excitation in the child that it was unable to bear, or of adults treating children with such coldness and spartan severity that it resulted in normal needs for warmth and tenderness exceeding the given possibilities of libidinal discharge and so evoking anxiety. He adds a third situation, which was described by Ferenczi in his seminal paper, 'Confusion of Tongues between the Adults and the Child' (1933), where the child, having been sexually excited by the adult and having openly shown it, is both rejected and subjected to severe moral reproof by the adult.

From this, Balint concludes that the therapeutic aim with these mistrustful patients is that they 'must learn in the course of treatment to be able again to give themselves up to love, to pleasure, to enjoyment, as fiercely and innocently as they were able to do in their earliest childhood' (1952a: 162). He discusses the technical processes required and introduces a new technical concept. Freud had written in 'Remembering, Repeating and Working-through' (1914) that the aim of the analytic work was to enable the patient to remember, and that this required some repetition or acting-out. Freud had suggested that the patient reproduced everything from the reservoirs of repressed material that had already permeated his general character – his inhibitions and disadvantageous attitudes of mind, which constituted his pathological traits of character. Balint adds that it is not only the pathological traits but all his traits of character that are displayed, as the patient could only behave as he really is. As these traits are analysed in their varied manifestations, it becomes clear that they are directed against the anxiety 'of full surrender, against the unbearable excitation: as this becomes conscious the situation in childhood usually also comes to light where the child's trust was betrayed' (1952a: 163).

Unfortunately, this coming to light in itself rarely results in change and Balint believes that in spite of the fact that the patient is helped to realize that he is no longer a child and that the analyst does not behave like the original adults, the change does not occur as the amount of excitation, the degree of the tension, is actually determined by the patient himself. Balint was then thinking in economic terms of amounts of excitation and tension bearable by the patient, and the task of the analyst was to help the patient achieve an optimal degree of tension as a result of which outbursts of affect occurred together with the appearance of fragments of memory not previously accessible to consciousness. He does not describe what his revision of technique consisted of; he himself states that 'without clinical examples, any discussion of technique is useless' (1952a: 164). It is unfortunate that often in his writings Balint does not give clinical examples to

17

illustrate his concepts, and this does tend to lessen the possibilities for the reader to understand his position fully.

Balint then describes that, together with an outburst of affect and the recovery of forgotten memories, a *new beginning* results. By this term he means 'a change in the behaviour, more exactly in the libido structure, of the patient . . . he still has to learn anew to be able to love innocently, unconditionally, as only children can love. This dropping of condition I call the new beginning' (1952a: 165). He gives the examples of one patient holding the analyst's finger in her hand; of another patient bringing a series of dreams day by day in which she was a child becoming older in successive dreams and doing nothing but love, with her different ways of loving repeating her whole development.

This, though, is then followed by an

> almost insatiable longing to repeat again and again such newly begun infantile manifestations of love. After this dies down, which only rarely takes any considerable time, the anxiety disappears and the patient is able to recognize and accept her newly begun wishes and either realize them in reality or renounce them.
>
> (1952a: 166)

This new beginning is repeated in various ways, and Balint equates this with the process of 'working-through' as described by Freud.

This account of these various processes will be seen as the forerunner of his future writing on the topic of therapeutic regression, which culminates in *The Basic Fault*. In this description is the origin of the process that thirty-six years later he calls *benign regression*, and in the brief reference to 'almost insatiable longings' he hints at the other type of regression, *malignant regression*.

Balint briefly considers the notion of character, and suggests that it 'controls the relation of man to the objects of his love and hate possibilities . . . it always means a more or less extensive limitation of love and hate possibilities . . . it means a limitation of the capacity for love and enjoyment' (1952a: 169). At the time of the writing of this paper in 1932, it was a controversial issue whether the analyst should attempt to alter the patient's character or not, and Balint with this discussion of technique and character is expressing the view that character analysis is both necessary and essential. This is the view that has later become universally accepted in treatment and training.

His paper in 1934 on 'The Final Goal of Psychoanalytic Treatment' is based partly on the arguments and views described in the previous paper on new beginning, and partly on the arguments which are to be set out more extensively and cogently in his next paper on the pre-genital organizations of the libido. This is one of Balint's seminal papers, written in

1935, and is entitled 'Critical Notes on the Theory of the Pregenital Organizations of the Libido'. It deals with the problem of 'the development of object-relations i.e. the development of love' (1935b: 51). The fact that he describes the development of object relations in terms of love, or libido, and not in terms of hate or destructiveness being an equal to love, is a theme that runs through all his thinking. He steadfastly maintains that the development of hate is always secondary to that of love and is not a primary drive in its right. It arises from experiences of frustration and separation. Of the British object relations school, only Fairbairn takes a similar position but in his own different theoretical framework.

The paper is devoted to the development of sexual object relations, and he intentionally does not discuss the changing instinctual sexual aims of oral, anal, urethral, genital, and other forms of gratification. He notes:

> However deeply we are able to penetrate with our analytic technique and observations into the history of a man's life, we have always, without exception, found object-relations. Auto-erotic forms of gratification were either harmless play, or they already represented compromise formations. They were revealed in analysis as mechanisms of consolation for, or of defence against, objects which had been lost or had led the child into severe conflicts. The same is true of the phenomena of so-called pregenital love, such as 'anal-sadistic' or 'phallic' love, and also of the 'negative Oedipus complex'. They are unimportant and harmless or, if of importance, then to be analysed and resolved. . . . I do not enquire why oral, and, urethral genital etc. forms of gratification appear in the development and what they signify, but confine my problem to the question *why the attitude of the individual to his environment and especially to his love-objects changes*, and what are the causes of the various forms of object-relations which we describe as oral, anal, phallic, genital, narcissistic, etc., love.
>
> (1935b: 59)

Balint held, following Ferenczi in *Thalassa*, that object relations predominate even in the deepest layers of the mind, and that in the end phase of deep analytic work, at the phase of the 'new beginning', the nature of this first object relation is expressed quite clearly:

> *The person in question does not love, but wishes to be loved. This passive wish is certainly sexual, libidinous.* The demand that these wishes shall be gratified by the environment is absolutely unproblematical and is often expressed quite vehemently with great displays of energy, almost as if it were a matter of life and death. The aim of all these wishes does not, however, correspond to what one generally means by sensual or erotic, but rather what Freud has called tender,

aim-inhibited. Non-gratification calls forth passionate reactions; gratification, on the other hand, only a quiet, tranquil sense of well-being.

(1935b: 61)

This primary tendency is called '*passive object-love*', a term introduced by Ferenczi, and is described as 'I shall be loved always, everywhere, in every way, my whole body, my whole being – without any criticism, without the slightest effort on my part – [this] is the final aim of all erotic striving' (1935b: 63). This primary tendency is retained throughout life and the attaining of it is achieved in roundabout ways; one way is via narcissism on the basis that 'if the world does not love me enough, I have to love and gratify myself' (1935b: 63). The other way is via 'active object-love', on the basis that 'we love and gratify our partner in order to be loved and gratified by him in return' (1935b: 66).

In his formulation of these two ways of re-achieving a passive object-love, Balint puts forward two important new psychoanalytical concepts. The first concerns the theory of narcissism. Balint demonstrates that there are several inconsistencies in the theory of primary narcissism, which leads him to suggest that the theory should be discarded in favour of primary object relationships and that narcissism is always a secondary phenomenon. This antedates the similar change in Melanie Klein's views on primary narcissism, since in 1936, Joan Riviere in her paper on the Kleinian position 'On the Genesis of Psychical Conflict in Earliest Infancy' given to the Vienna Psychoanalytical Society was using the concept of primary narcissism prior to object-relatedness: 'These two counterparts represent the aims and significance of the projection and introjection focuses, which develop out of primary narcissism as external objects begin to be perceived' (1952: 52).

The second new concept concerns the nature of the active object-love. He writes:

Others, however – and they form the vast majority – can reach the aim of the 'passive object-love' only by roundabout ways. Education enforces, even devises, these by-paths. If the child is offered too little, it invests its auto-erotism, hitherto practised in a playful way, with its whole libido, becomes narcissistic or aggressive or both. If it gets something it becomes, as it were, moulded by the gratification received. The successive stages of development so frequently and regularly found – anal-sadistic, phallic and finally genital object-relations – have not a biological but a cultural basis. As you see I have left out the oral relation. Purposely, for I cannot make culture, i.e. education, solely responsible for this.

(Balint 1935b: 63)

Looked at in this way, the pregenital object-relations, the pregenital forms of love, appear in another light. They can no longer be explained biologically, but must be considered, to use perhaps a rather strong expression, as artifacts, i.e. we must make society in general, or the individual educator in question, responsible for them. Moreover, our clinical therapy has always acted as if this were an acknowledged fact.

(1935b: 66)

He then goes on to add:

Thus, and I mean it quite seriously, if children could be properly brought up, they would not have to struggle through the complicated forms of pregenital object-relations which are only forced upon them. . . . But today I cannot visualise clearly this development from passive object-love with its tender sexual aim, to active object-love with its genital sensual aims. All the less because the origin of passionateness, of sensual orgastic lust, is not clear to me.

(1935b: 67)

Balint is differentiating the pre-genital aims of sexuality from the varieties of pre-genital object-relational organizations and is claiming that the latter are not directly related to the former in a biologically determined manner. The pre-genital aims themselves are biologically determined, but the way that these are incorporated into the object-relational organizations is determined by the environment – that is, culture and education. This interesting line of investigation into the relationship between these two lines is not, however, continued in his further papers, where he concentrates on object relationships and not on pre-genital phases. However, with this differentiation of the development of human relations from the development of sexual aims towards objects, Balint is describing a situation which was later to be developed in his own way by Winnicott (1963). Winnicott differentiates between the 'object-mother' and the 'environment-mother', describing 'the environment-mother who receives all that can be called affection and sensuous co-existence; it is the object-mother who becomes the target for excited experience backed by crude instinct-tension' (p. 76). This resembles Balint's dual development lines, but Winnicott relates the development of the capacity for concern to the coming together in the infant's mind of the object-mother and environment-mother, rather than considering the effects of culture and education on these two lines as Balint has done.

In his next paper, 'Eros and Aphrodite' (1936b), he turns to the other topic that he specifically excluded from 'Pregenital Organizations of the Libido', the development of sexual aims, of the acquisition of pleasure, of erotism, of sensual orgastic lust. It is principally an examination of the difference between fore-pleasure and end-pleasure in libidinal experiences. He suggests that they are two separate modes of experiencing pleasure, akin but fundamentally different, and believes that this hypothesis is supported (1) by the fact that end-pleasure seems to be designed to make adult humans more immune from anxiety, and (2) that perverts derive no gratification from their actual perverse activity other than powerful excitation; relief comes subsequently from genital masturbation or coitus. In this, Balint differs from Ferenczi, whose theory of amphimixis postulated that end-pleasure was the sum total of the component instinct mechanisms of fore-pleasure. Balint thinks that the function of fore-pleasure is comparatively simple and seems to be a primary attribute of living beings, whereas end-pleasure, orgasm, is a new acquisition in the history of the race and is complicated, since it is composed of two opposite tendencies of dealing with excitation. There is an uncoordinated chronic spasm of movement, together with a constricting tonic spasm; both, being experienced together, are all but traumatic in intensity. He suggests that the psychological 'strength of the ego' 'may be measured by the maximum tension or excitation which it can tolerate without disturbance, and, where conditions are fairly normal, the only excitation which approximates to the maximum in adults is the excitation before and during orgasm' (1936b: 86).

This is the last paper in which Balint gives us his ideas on psychobiological and instinctual lines of development, until we reach his ideas on the subject of thrills in his later book, *Thrills and Regressions* (1959a).

His next paper, one of the most important, develops the theme of primary object-love from his 1935 paper. It is entitled 'Early Developmental States of the Ego: Primary Object-love' (1937b). He starts with a description of the two theoretical views on infantile development as exemplified by the London school of Melanie Klein and the Viennese school of Freud. At this time, because of the theoretical differences and controversies between these two schools and in the interests of possible reconciliation, there had been an exchange of papers between the two societies. Joan Riviere of the London school had read a paper 'On the Genesis of Psychical Conflict in Earliest Infancy' to the Vienna Society in May 1936, and Robert Waelder of Vienna had read a paper on the identical topic to the British Society in November 1936. The outcome, however, effected no reconciliation between the two schools of thought, and Balint suggests that possibly a third way, that of the Budapest Society, might help to bridge some of the gap between the two other theories on the basis of new and fresh clinical material. This material derives from considering the formal elements in the analytic situation as phenomena of transference, and that in this way there is a possibility of obtaining valuable data about the individual history of patients. It must be remembered that although the analysis of the formal elements in the transference–counter-transference relationship in the analytic setting, is nowadays standard analytic technique, at that time this was certainly not the case. Ferenczi was one of the pioneers of this form of investigation, and when he died in 1933, his work was carried on by his successors, Michael Balint, Alice Balint and Imre Hermann.

What are these new clinical data?

I found that at times, when the analytic work had advanced fairly deeply, my patients expected and often even demanded certain primitive gratifi-cations, mainly from their analyst but also from their environment. If I kept strictly to the rule of analytic passivity, i.e. if these desires for gratification were frustrated automatically by my passivity, phenomena appeared which corresponded in all their essential features to the conception of the infant as put forward by the London analysts. Loss of security, the feeling of being worthless, despair, deeply bitter disappointment, the feeling that one would never be able to trust anyone, etc. Mixed with these came most venomous aggression, wildest sadistic phantasies and orgies depicting the most cunning tortures and humiliation for the analyst. Then again fear of retaliation, the most complete contriteness, because one had spoilt for ever the hope of being loved by the analyst or even merely to be treated by him with interest and kindness. . . . If, however – warned by the experiences I have quoted – I later permitted the satisfaction of those modest wishes, we simply went from the frying pan into the fire. An almost manic state broke out. The patients became over-blissful; they wanted nothing but to experience again and again the satisfaction of those wishes. All the symptoms disappeared; the patients felt super-healthy as long as they felt sure of obtaining immediately on demand the satisfaction of these extremely important wishes . . . this state very closely resembles that of an addiction or of a severe perversion, even in its lability. At the first serious dissatisfaction or considerable delay of the gratification the whole structure of this enraptured blissfulness breaks down and abruptly the mood changes into the form described previously of despair, hatred and fear of retaliation. . . . What are these dangerous wishes in reality? Rather innocent, naïve one would say. A kind word from the analyst, the permission to call him by his first name or be called by him by one's first name; to be able to see him also outside the analytical session, to borrow something or to get a present from him even if it be quite insignificant, etc. Very often these wishes do not go further than to be able to touch the analyst, to cling to him, or to be touched or stroked by him.

(Balint 1937b: 96–8)

He notices that the two essential qualities of these wishes are that they are always directed towards an object, and that they never go beyond the level of fore-pleasure. From this, it follows that only the environment could satisfy those wishes, and that the satisfaction could best be described as a tranquil, quiet sense of well-being. If these wishes, however, remain unsatisfied, the reaction would be of the stormy and vehement kind already described. From these premises, he argues that these phenomena are not simply primary reactions but that they already have a history in the patient's development and this involves the developments from the state of primary passive object-love as described in the earlier paper ('Critical Notes', 1935); from primary-love, one detour is to narcissism, and the other, to active object-love.

Balint sums up his researches so far as follows:

1 The phase of primary or primitive object-love must occur very early in life.
2 This phase is unavoidable and all later object relations can be traced back to it.
3 This form of object relation is not linked to any of the erotogenic zones, 'a fact of paramount importance, and I hope that through this strict discrimination it will be possible to disentangle the hopeless confusion brought about by equating the development of instinctual aims with the development of instinctual object relations' (1952b: 101). (He does not, however, develop this line of thought in his further writings.)
4 The biological basis of this primary object relation is the instinctual interdependence of mother and child. 'The two are dependent on each other but at the same time they are tuned to each other; each of them satisfies himself by the other without the compulsion of paying regard to the other. Indeed, what is good for the one is right for the other. This biological interdependence in the dual unit has been considered hitherto only very superficially; e.g. we thought we had explained it, from the mother's side, by a narcissistic identification with her child' (1937b: 102).
5 This intimate relation is severed by our civilization much too early. Consequences of this early severance are the tendency to cling, to discontentment, and to insatiable greed in children.
6 If the instinctual desire is satisfied in time, there is the tranquil sense of well-being. If frustrated, there are the extremely vehement reactions, and he suggests that possibly only such misunderstood and hence misinterpreted environmental influences can cause reactively in the child symptoms of insatiable cravings.

As an aside here, it is worth noticing that in this paper of 1937, from his description of the formal aspects of the analytic setting, Balint comes to conclusions arrived at by later observational studies. He is the forerunner of Winnicott's later dictum that there is no such thing as a baby without a mother, and the forerunner of the conclusions of much later infant–baby observational research, such as that of John Bowlby (1969, 1973, 1980) and Daniel Stern (1985), with their concepts of mutual attachment and emotional attunement between mother and infant.

Balint believes that one of the main sources of the polemical differences between Vienna and London at that time was the hypothesis of primary narcissism, and he devoted considerable space to marshalling clinical observations and theoretical arguments to counter this hypothesis. Balint frequently returns to the arguments against primary narcissism in later papers and, most cogently and pungently, in a chapter on this topic in his last book *The Basic Fault* (1968). It is almost as though for Balint, the establishment of arguments against primary narcissism was as important as the establishment of arguments in favour of the existence of the unconscious was for Freud. I shall defer consideration of these arguments until we examine this later book. Nevertheless, to return to the polemic of the paper, he believes:

> The English felt that they were right in emphasizing the insatiability of the children. However, their thinking got arrested here and they could not go on to view the infantile situation as an instinctual interdependence of mother and child. And the reason for this inability is the fact that they – in the same way as the Viennese – cling desperately to the hypothesis of primary narcissism. This hypothesis bars the assumption of any relation to external objects. To counter it the Londoners could do nothing but stress time and again their rather one-sided clinical material about the aggressive phenomena showing the infantile dissatisfaction.
>
> (1952b: 103)

Today, of course, Kleinians have long dispensed with the theory of primary narcissism and so have many contemporary Freudians, yet the differences between these two schools still persist in spite of this. Balint's hopeful and optimistic prediction concerning these adverse effects of the theory of primary narcissism has not stood the test of time.

The other significant aspect of this paper is his discussion of the clinical effects of gratification or non-gratification of desires and wishes. This is to be one of the cornerstones of his future clinical and theoretical contributions to the study of therapeutic regression in psychoanalysis, culminating in his formulations set out in *The Basic Fault*.

'Love for the Mother and Mother Love' (1939) is a paper written not by Michael but by Alice Balint, and he has included it in his 1952 volume on the basis of their 'intertwining development'. She relates the earliest form of love to an archaic object-relation lacking any sense of reality, but from which what we are wont to call love develops directly under the influence of reality. . . . The archaic love without reality sense is the form of the love of the id, which persists as such throughout life, while the social reality-based form of love represents the manner of loving of the ego.

(1952a: 126)

This archaic love, which was first described as passive object-love, is now described as primary object-love, since active tendencies in the infant are seen to play a paramount role, and Balint henceforth drops the passive nomenclature in all future references to the term. The new emphasis on the activity of the infant from the beginning is, as previously mentioned, the forerunner of much of the most recent work on mother–infant observational research.

Balint, in his next paper, 'Strength of the Ego and its Education' (1938), concerns himself with the role of learning in psychoanalytic treatment and he criticizes it from the point of view of the structural approach. He suggests that

psychoanalytic pedagogy has been chiefly a pedagogy of the super-ego, and its main problem was to find out what type of educational method, and applied in what degree of intensity, was best fitted to relieve an optimal formation of the superego.

(1952a: 209)

He believes this to be due to the fact that psychoanalytical theory had been largely developed on the basis of the study of obsessional neurosis and depression, and that the problem of hysteria had been increasingly neglected. Obsessional neurosis and depression are viewed as largely a psychology of the superego, whereas hysteria usually concerns bodily functioning where 'the ego is, above all, a body ego and the problems that arise here make manifold encroachments on to the field of biology, taking "the mysterious leap into the organic".'

In later papers, he develops this theme of superego pedagogy in relation to problems of the training of psychoanalysts, and also develops the theme of the body-ego and its influences when, in *The Basic Fault*, he puts forward the view of the therapeutic value of the non-verbal components of the object relationship between patient and analyst as one of the agents of psychic change, as against the view that only verbal transference interpretations, particularly of Strachey's mutative transference variety, are the agent of psychic change. As Balint put it in this paper, 'education of the ego is not a technical measure specially to be employed during the treatment; it is rather an immanent component of the analysis' (1952a: 211).

'On Transference and Counter-transference' (1939) was written in collaboration with his wife, Alice, and was one of the first papers to be written on the subject of the counter-transference. Previously, in a paper, 'On Transference of Emotions' (1933), he had equated counter-transference with the analyst's own transference to the patient, but now in 1939 he extends it to include everything in the analytic setting, from his own person down to the arrangement of the cushions on the couch, which reveals something of the personality of the analyst. A decade later, in his paper on 'Changing Therapeutical Aims and Techniques in Psycho-analysis' (1949), he uses the term synonymously with phrases such as 'correct analytical behaviour' and 'proper handling of the transference situation'. It has now come to mean for him the total professional attitude in all dimensions of the analyst towards the patient. This view is only one of the many on the nature of the counter-transference that have been put forward in the literature.

He suggests on the basis of the statistics published by the different psychoanalytical institutes in the 1930s that, on the whole, the same percentage of successful and unsuccessful outcomes of treatment are obtained by all the differing psychoanalytic techniques. He wondered 'why then the heated discussions and the comparative intolerance in matters of technique?' (1952a: 219), and suggested that it was an instance of the social phenomenon termed 'the narcissistic overvaluation of small differences'. This disagreement has indeed remained remarkably persistent over the years and shows no signs of abating.

Balint returns to object relationships in a short paper 'On Genital Love' (1947), and introduces the concept of '*work of conquest*'.

> In order to win a loving and lovable genital object and to keep it for good, nothing could be taken for granted as happened in oral love; a permanent, never-relaxing, exacting reality testing must be kept up all the time. This might be called the work of conquest (conversely for the subject this means an exacting piece of adaptation to his object). It is most exacting in the initial stages of a relation, but in a milder form must be maintained unwaveringly throughout the whole duration. In other words, the two partners must always be in harmony.
>
> (1952a: 135)

The reward for bearing the strain of this work is the possibility of regressing periodically for some happy moments to an infantile step of reality testing, to the 'mystic union' of the genital orgasm. This idea of harmony between objects is developed further in his later writings.

'On Love and Hate' (1951) examines the various attempts to explain the characteristics of primitive and adult love and hate and he puts forward his own view of hatred. He starts from the premise that there are primitive and mature forms of love, whereas hatred is always primitive. He believes that the various attempts to explain the differences between primitive and adult love complement each other rather than being mutually exclusive, and cites factors such as the weakness of the ego, undeveloped or faulty reality testing, strong innate sadistic tendencies, splitting processes, strong narcissistic tendencies, depressive fears, oral greed and despondent omnipotence to explain the differences. In primitive object relationships, however, he believes that 'only one partner is entitled to make demands, the other is treated as an object, albeit as an instinct or love-object' and 'the basis of all such relationships is faulty reality testing, either still undeveloped (in infants) or stunted (in adults)' (1952a: 146). The change to mutual love comes with the previously described work of conquest.

Where does he place hatred?

> In my opinion, hate is the last remnant, the desire of, and the defence against, the primitive object-love (or the dependent archaic love). This means that we hate people who, though very important to us, do not love us and refuse to become our co-operative partners despite our best efforts to win their affection.
>
> (1952a: 148)

The importance of this is that, for Balint, hatred is always secondary to love and as previously mentioned, only Fairbairn, among the British object relations school, has a similar view of this relationship, although he does not follow Balint in the belief in primary object love. Balint thinks that hatred is the outcome of the various factors, such as weakness of the ego, undeveloped reality testing and so on which are listed above, and that this would affect the outcome of all analyses. He suggests that various outcomes of analysis may arise:

> in some cases the result of treatment will be health behind barriers of hatred, a costly but not-too-bad protection against the wish to regress. In other cases, the result will be a perpetual dependent identification, defending by idealisation the object against our hatred. And lastly, in favourable cases, the lasting marks of this fateful primary object relation, of the primary transference, may amount only to *unforgettable memories, sweet and painful at the same time.*
>
> (1952a: 156)

Why does Balint insist on the secondary reactive defensive nature of hatred? He does not follow Ferenczi in this respect since, although Ferenczi believed that hate could be reactive, he also believed that it was a primary destructive drive in its own right as described by Freud. Presumably his theory derives from his clinical experiences of providing small gratifications to patients in regressed states and obtaining a benign hateless reaction

28

instead of the hatred-filled response to frustrations. Under these benign conditions it seems that there is only a quiet innocent love in the clinical atmosphere; hence the secondary nature of hatred. However, my own experience of such states is that sometimes in the next session or after a dream, one can detect signs that the state was not as benign as it seemed, but represented a defensive manoeuvre against split-off and denied persecutory states (see 1952a: 166). The state of affairs does not seem to be as simple as Balint suggests.

Another of his most important papers, that on 'Changing Therapeutical Aims and Techniques in Psychoanalysis' (1949), is a critical account of the theory of technique and its changes, starting from 1922 when he began to practise psychoanalysis. According to Balint, at first the aim of therapy was to overcome the patient's resistance, to remove infantile amnesia and to make the unconscious conscious. The unconscious then meant only the repressed, infantile amnesia, and the Oedipal situation. With the coming of the structural theory of the mind, the aim changed and became the replacement of id by ego; to help the patient to repair the faulty ego structure; and to help the patient abandon costly defence mechanisms and develop less costly ones. The older or dynamic approach was more concerned with content, with the id, and the newer, structural approach with defensive structures of the ego and superego. Both formulations were, however, concerned only with the individual and not with the object, the physiological or biological bias, as Balint terms it.

A new orientation in technique now focused not only on the contents of free associations and on the detection of habitual defence mechanisms, but also on the formal elements of the patient's behaviour, such as changing facial expressions, ways of lying on the couch, ways of associating and so on. He believes that these elements are closely linked with the patient's character and are part and parcel of the patient's transference towards the world and, particularly in the analytic situation, towards his analyst.

> They have to be regarded as phenomena of some kind of object-relation – often of a primitive type – which has been revived in (or perhaps by) the psychoanalytical situation. The consequent study of these formal elements of the patient's behaviour was, in my opinion, the main factor that brought about a fundamental change, indeed a very great improvement, in our technical skills. This new orientation in our technique aims, first and foremost, at understanding and interpreting every detail of the patient's transference in terms of object-relations.
>
> ('Changing Therapeutical Aims and Technique', 1952a: 225)

He described this as the 'object-relation bias', in contrast with the previous 'physiological or biological bias'.

These two forms of bias, he postulates, occur in conjunction with a discrepancy between our technique and our theory of psychopathology.

> Our theory has been mainly based on the study of pathological forms which use internalization extensively and have only weakly cathected object-relations; our technique was invented and has been mainly developed when working with pathological forms such as hysteria, sexual disorders, character neurosis, all of which have strongly cathected object-relations. This, however, is only natural, as our true field of study is the psychoanalytical situation, a situation where relations to an object – admittedly a very peculiar object – are of overwhelming importance. A good deal of internal contradiction and of conflicting tendencies in psychoanalysis becomes understandable if we always bear in mind this double origin of our technique and theory.
>
> ('Changing Therapeutical Aims and Technique', 1952a: 227)

He pays tribute to John Rickman's ideas (1951) of one-body psychology, two-body, three-body, and multi-body psychology, where each psychology should have its own field of studies and develop its own language of technical terms and concepts. These ideas would include Balint's previously mentioned observation that psychoanalytic theory is almost entirely based on a one-body psychology derived from its study of obsessional states and melancholia, whereas the language of technique is almost entirely based on a two-body psychology. He continues, 'what we need now is a theory that would give us a good description of the development of object-relations comparable to, but independent of, our present, biologising, theory of the development of instincts' ('Changing Therapeutical Aims and Technique', 1952a: 230).

Here he discusses Melanie Klein's theory of the development of object relations. She created new terms,

> such as part-objects, which may be good or bad, can be split off or reintegrated, destroyed or repaired, introjected or projected, and so on. If we accept that introjection and projection, splitting etc. mean some structural changes in the mind, then Mrs Klein's theories can be regarded as an attempt at relating changes in the object-relations to structural changes in the mind. Obviously this is a very important step, and most likely is the transition between the old theories and the new ones demanded by me.
>
> ('Changing Therapeutical Aims and Technique', 1952a: 231)

For this coming new theory, he thinks that the most important field of investigation would be the analyst's behaviour in the psychoanalytic situation, the analyst's contribution to the creating and maintaining of the psychoanalytic situation. He means by this not only the giving of the correct interpretation to the patient, but also the appreciation by the analyst of how much and what kind of frustrations and satisfactions were required by both the patient and the analyst in order to keep the tension in the analytical situation as near optimal as possible. He thinks that the language of the analyst – by which he meant his set of technical terms, his concepts, his models, his frames of reference, which are used to convey inter-pretations – is extremely important in the development and shaping of these tensions. The different languages of different analysts need observing and studying in the development of the new theory of object relations. In addition to this, he thinks that the creation of a proper atmosphere by the analyst for the patient is necessary in order to help the patient to open up. These concepts of the analytic language, of the consideration of the necessary frustrations and satisfactions, and of the action of a proper atmosphere, are considerably developed, and integrated in his later writings, particularly in *The Basic Fault*.

In his contribution to the issue of the *International Journal of Psycho-Analysis* to honour the seventieth birthday of Melanie Klein, a long-standing friend of his, which is entitled 'New Beginning and the Paranoid and Depressive Syndromes' (1952b), Balint is concerned to show how some of her ideas on human development coincide with his own observations and theories. He describes again the late phase of some analyses, first described in his 1932 paper, 'Character Analysis and New Beginning', and developed in his 1937 paper on 'Primary Object-love'. In this phase, in a mutually trusting atmosphere, the patient desires certain simple gratifications from the analyst, which, if acceded to, give a tranquil sense of well-being and the possibility of a new beginning, the capacity for unsuspicious, trusting, self-abandoned relaxation of defences. However, this does not necessarily happen and the patient becomes addictively greedy for gratification, never having enough; if the gratifications are frustrated, an overwhelming flood of sadistic behaviour ensues. This creates great difficulties for the analyst in attempting to steer an even course, but if this is successfully negotiated, the new beginning might ensue.

His clinical experience shows him that before a phase of new beginning could develop, the patient has to go through a phase in which his paranoid attitudes have to be relinquished to some extent, and accompanied by the recognition that they were grossly exaggerated. This is followed by a further phase in which a certain amount of depression has to be accepted as an inevitable necessary condition of ordinary life. The sequence of phases therefore is paranoid state → depressive state → archaic object-love of new beginning, and this corresponds with Klein's sequence of positions, paranoid-schizoid and depressive, as postulated for infantile development.

31

If this sequence is correct, Balint thinks he would have to give up his own theory of primary (archaic) object-love being the first stage of development.

He, however, argues against this sequence in human development terms. First, he points out that the paranoid and depressive states both contain many narcissistic features, and according to Balint (and according to the later Klein), narcissism is always a secondary state and never primary. Second, he maintains that both the paranoid and depressive states are fraught with anxieties that may be lessened, whereas primary object-love contains no inherent anxiety. For both reasons, he prefers that the earliest stage be that of primary object-love, rather than the paranoid–schizoid position postulated by Klein, and that this archaic object-love should be considered as a nodal point from which all later developments radiate. He describes four of these developments:

1 narcissism (if I am not loved in the way I want it, I must love myself);
2 the paranoid and depressive attitudes, interlinked, and each able to be used as a defence against the other;
3 anal-sadistic object-relations, due to educational influences;
4 adult sexuality and genital object-love.

('New Beginning and the Paranoid and the Depressive Syndromes', 1952b: 262–3)

With this description of the four phases of development of object relations arising from the nodal point of primary object-love, Balint gives his first coherent theory of the development of object relations. It is not until 1968, in the chapter on 'Primary Love' in his book *The Basic Fault* (1968), that he develops the theory further and gives a new version, particularly of the early stages, and this will be described in the chapter on *The Basic Fault* (pages 47–60 of this book). It is very possible that, had he lived, he might well have made further changes to his theory.

He realizes that there is no certain way of deciding this issue of the primacy of phases, and adds a further complication by wondering about the extent to which the analyst's techniques – that is his attitudes in the analytic situation, his theoretical expectations and orientation, his set of technical terms and so on – would also influence, and perhaps produce, the very phenomena that are being observed.

Lastly, Balint makes a short but important statement on 'the interrelation between the development of libidinous object-relations on the one hand and that of reality-testing on the other'. He remarks:

Primary, archaic object-relation needs hardly any reality-testing; there is no need to account for the object. A change is brought about by the experience of being frustrated or being compelled to wait for satisfaction by an indifferent, insufficiently considerate, or even hostile environment. This enforces upon the child a very primitive kind of reality testing, resulting in splitting the object into a frustrating bad, and into a gratifying good, part-object. Out of the former develop the hostile, persecutory or depressing objects, out of the latter – as a kind of reaction – formation or reparation – the phantasy of the idealized object.

(1952b: 262–3)

Here he is taking the view that in Klein's two positions, the paranoid-schizoid and the depressive, there is an intermingling of both unconscious phantasy elements and the reality perception of objects, rather than the emphasis being almost exclusively focused on the unconscious phantasies of the infant, which is Klein's viewpoint.

With this tribute to, and acknowledgement of, the work of Mrs Klein, Balint ends this book with its many lines of the development of important theoretical and technical issues in psychoanalysis up to 1952.

The main thrust throughout the book is that of the primacy of object relations. Balint's concept of the original relationship is that of primary active object-love, with hatred being a secondary phenomenon. The concept arose from observations of the clinical responses of certain types of regressed patients to relatively minor gratifications. A necessary corollary of the primacy of object-love was to call the concept of primary narcissism into question and show that all the clinical manifestations were secondary in nature. Primary object-love is regarded as a nodal point for further developments, leading in his first formulation to both narcissism and to active adult object-love. To these was added pre-genital object relations, and in his final formulation in this book, he adds paranoid and depressive attitudes. In later works, there will be further developments described from this nodal point.

Similarly, psychoanalytical technique is also examined from the view-point of object relations. Rather than concentrating on the patient and the patient's transference, Balint has followed the lead given by Ferenczi of investigating the analyst's contribution to the analytic situation. The counter-transference responses, the theoretical orientation, the technical terminology of the analyst are seen to influence, and perhaps produce, the very phenomena being observed in the analytic situation. This mutual interaction between patient and analyst as described here has today become the very centre of contemporary psychoanalytic technique and theory.

2

Problems of Human Pleasure and Behaviour
(1956)

This book, Balint's second, was published in 1957. It consists of a number of articles and reviews of a more general nature and does not set out to develop any particular themes in depth nor to develop any of the themes from his previous book other than peripherally. These articles and reviews were published in a variety of journals over the period 1923–56 and show Balint's interests and thinking over a wide variety of subjects. The book is divided into three sections, entitled 'The Individual and the Community', 'Clinical Problems' and 'Men and their Ideas'.

Balint had from early on in his career been concerned with the social aspects of psychoanalysis and was friendly with like-minded colleagues, such as Geza Roheim and Otto Fenichel, who constituted a left-wing, radical progressive group of the psychoanalysts in Budapest. These interests are evidenced in the topics selected in the first section on the individual and the community, and include 'Sex and Society' (1956); 'The Problem of Discipline' (1951a); 'The Adolescent's Fight against Masturbation' (1934a); 'The Psychological Problems of Growing Old' (1933a); 'On Punishing Offenders' (1951b); and 'Notes on the Dissolution of Object-representation in Modern Art' (1952d). The essays demonstrate a very extensive knowledge of cultural, artistic and social affairs, the product of the cultured intelligentsia of Central Europe. Interestingly, this section also includes a chapter on individual differences of behaviour in early infancy as evidenced by the sucking rhythms of bottle-fed infants, for which he devised a method to record them. He hoped by this to establish 'deeply rooted, innate, constitutional differences between different individuals' (1956a: 149); that is, something that is not determined by social factors in the environment. He believed that the importance of his findings was to show that these individual differences in sucking rhythms could be demonstrated in the very first days of life. This study in 1945 was used by him to obtain his PhD degree whilst he was working in Manchester, and this area of early bodily experiences was further developed in his next books, *Thrills and*

Regressions and *The Basic Fault*, where they constitute an important aspect of non-verbal experience for the individual. The non-verbal experience is of great theoretical and technical importance for Balint, particularly in considering the therapeutic potential both of interpretation and of object relationships.

The second part of the book is devoted to clinical problems, and includes essays on 'Contributions to Reality Testing' (1942); 'A Contribution on Fetishism' (1934); 'A Contribution to the Psychology of Menstruation' (1937a); 'Perversion or a Hysterical Symptom?' (1923), which was his very first psychoanalytical paper; 'Notes on Parapsychology and Parapsychological Healing'; and 'The Doctor, His Patient and the Illness' (1955b).

Balint was interested in the phenomenon of parapsychology, partly, probably, because of the interest taken in it by both Ferenczi and Freud. In his essay, Balint suggests that parapsychological phenomena may be produced by the patient if the analyst's mind is temporarily preoccupied with matters external to the analytic situation but is pretending that his interest and attention are really focused on the patient. The phenomenon, usually of telling the analyst something about the analyst where it would often have been impossible for the patient to acquire the information, will have the effect of therapeutically shocking the analyst into giving his full attention and interest again.

The paper, 'The Doctor, His Patient and the Illness', was later the title of Balint's perhaps most famous and internationally acclaimed book. It was published in the *Lancet*, the famous medical journal, in 1955 and was in fact the vehicle by which I first came to know and to meet him. The paper concerns his pioneering work with general medical practitioners which he carried out at the Tavistock Clinic, and its importance lies in the fact that it gives these doctors a new role in the understanding of their patients' emotional problems and behaviour. As I have already outlined in the introduction, his technical advance in this area was to introduce the concept of the doctor as being a most important drug for the patient, necessitating the determination of the dosage and frequency of this drug for therapeutic purposes. He introduced the importance of allowing the patient to complain in his own good time, and of the doctor allowing himself to experience his own emotions and phantasies in his relationship with the patient. This is, of course, a training for the doctor in using his own counter-transference reactions to the patient. He also introduced the concept of the apostolic function of the doctor, by which he meant his attitudes and responses to the patient's complaints together with his expectations of the patient. It can be seen that in these ideas of counter-transference emotional reactions and apostolic functions of the general practitioner, Balint is using his concept of the term 'counter-transference', as described in his technical psychoanalytic paper of 1949, where it means the totality of the analyst's analytical behaviour and professional attitude towards the patient. The insights of the analytic discipline are being used to facilitate the practice of the physician's discipline.

At the end of this essay, Balint adds a postscript in which, almost as an afterthought, he introduces one of his most important concepts, that of the basic fault. He writes:

> Throughout this address, I have used 'illness' in the same sense as it is used in general medicine. . . . If I am right, psychoanalysis is about to develop a new conception which may be called 'basic illness' or perhaps 'basic fault' in the biological structure of the individual, involving in varying degrees both his mind and his body. The origin of this basic fault, according to this theory, may be traced back to a considerable discrepancy in the early formative years or possibly months of the individual between his own needs and the care and nursing available at the relevant times. This creates a state of deficiency whose consequences are only partly reversible. Although the individual may achieve a good or even a very good adjustment, the vestiges of his early experiences remain and contribute to a large extent to what is called his constitution, his individuality, or his character make-up both in the psychological and the biological sense. The cause of this early discrepancy may be congenital, i.e. the infant's needs may be too exacting, or may be environmental, such as insufficient, careless, haphazard, over-anxious, over-protecting, or only un-understanding care. Should this theoretical approach prove correct, then all the pathological states of later years, the 'clinical illnesses' must be considered as symptoms or exacerbations of the 'basic illness', brought about by the various crises in the development, both external and internal, psychological or biological, of the individual.
>
> (1956a: 219–20)

This important new concept will be developed further in his later book with this title, and it will then be associated with the subtitle, 'Therapeutic Aspects of Regression', where regression in analysis is the vehicle by which the phenomena of the basic fault may be reached and often ameliorated.

The last section of the book, 'Men and their Ideas', is devoted to brief reviews of the work of various people such as I. P. Pavlov and his work on conditioned reflexes (1927); Sandor Ferenczi (1933) and (1948); Marquis de Sade (1954c); Geza Roheim (1954b); Szondi and his 'Triebdiagnostik' (1948c); and finally a critical review of W.R. Fairbairn's book, *Psychoanalytic Studies of the Personality*, published in 1953, called 'Pleasure, Object and Libido' (1956). Fairbairn had put forward an extensive new model of endopsychic structure to replace Freud's tripartite mode of ego, id and superego, and had also maintained an important new thesis that libido is not pleasure-seeking as Freud had maintained, but was object-seeking. Fairbairn had suggested in his book that

1 libido is essentially object seeking;
2 erotogenic zones are not themselves primary determinants of libidinal aims, but channels mediating the primary object-seeking aims of the ego;
3 any theory of ego development that is to be satisfactory must be conceived in terms of relationships with objects, and in particular relationships with objects which have been internalized, during early life under the pressure of deprivation and frustration.

(Fairbairn 1952: 162)

Balint maintained strongly that the phenomena observable in the analytic situations on which Fairbairn had based his theoretical conclusions could never be properly or fully representative of early human development, of the relationship between mother and infant. It is inherent in the analytic situation that there can never be any of the cruder physical and basic instinctual satisfactions and gratifications in the analytical situation and these needs can only be frustrated, whereas these gratifications and satisfactions are essential in mother–infant encounters. Balint argued that because of this basic difference, all psychoanalytical theories of development based entirely on the analytic situation must be one-sided and limited. He suggested that Fairbairn's three points could be retranslated into a two-person psychology language:

1 Only little fully gratifying pleasure is observable in the analytic situation, especially pleasure of the high-intensity type; but in his search for some gratification there is an almost inexhaustible urge in the patient to develop new and even newer object-relations to his, on the whole, frustrating analyst.
2 The role of erotogenic zones in the analytic situation is negligible as compared with the very great urge to develop object-relations to the analyst.
3 The patient's development, as it may be observed in the analytic situation, is under the constant and overwhelming influence of the internalized frustrating and depriving analyst.

(1956a: 289)

3

Thrills and Regressions (1959)

With this book, published in 1959, Balint continues with his exploration of the development of primitive attitudes and object relationships in his patients in the course of the analytic situation. As the title suggests, it is mainly concerned with the related phenomena of thrills and regressions, both of which can be readily experienced not only in analysis but also in everyday life situations, the most common being the experiences that people have at fun-fairs.

In his Introduction, he gives an account of his objections to using the term 'oral' to describe everything primitive:

> Practically all our technical terms describing the early period of mental life have been derived from objective phenomena and/or subjective experiences of the 'oral' sphere; as, for instance: greed, incorporation, introjection, internalization, part-objects; destruction by sucking, chewing and biting; projection according to the pattern of spitting and vomiting; etc. Sadly enough, we have almost completely neglected to enrich our understanding of these very early, very primitive phenomena by creating theoretical notions and coining technical terms using the experiences, imagery, and implications of other spheres. Such spheres are among others: feelings of warmth, rhythmic noises and movements, subdued nondescript humming, the irresistible and overwhelming effects of tastes and smells, of close bodily contact, of tactile and muscle sensations especially in the hands, and the undeniable power of any and all of these for provoking and allaying anxieties and suspicions, blissful contentment, and desperate loneliness.
>
> (1959a: 12)

This constitutes a powerful argument in support of his thesis, first put forward in the book *Primary Love and Psychoanalytic Technique* (1952), that the development of object relationships and the development of instinctual drives, though continuously influencing each other, are fundamentally different processes. Many of the non-oral primitive phenomena that have just been delineated can hardly be described as instinctual in aim, but they are certainly somatic modalities vital to object relationships. Their importance is now being demonstrated in modern infant–mother research, and here again, Balint's thinking has been ahead of his time.

He now proceeds to discuss the topic of fun-fairs and thrills, which must be one of the most unusual venues for a psychoanalytical investigation. He considers the various traditional pleasures found at most fun-fairs and concentrates his attention on two of them; these are the 'aggressive pleasures, such as throwing or shooting at things, smashing things up, etc., and pleasures connected with dizziness, vertigo, impairment or loss of stability, such as swings, roundabouts, switchbacks' (1959a: 19). The aggressive pleasures represent opportunities for regressive behaviour, offering satisfaction for primitive destructive and aggressive instincts. He notes that this destructive and aggressive behaviour is not only accepted by the environment but is also usually rewarded with some prize, together with the environment rejoicing in the destruction. Balint thinks that because the environment really does this, and because this type of object relationship is satisfying to both parties, this behaviour cannot readily be accounted for in the usual theoretical framework other than his own concept of primary love, where there is complete harmony, complete identity of wishes and satisfactions between the two partners. Because of this, he suggests that fun-fairs offer possibilities for limited regression to this early phase of human relationship.

Thrills are the pleasures associated with swings, roundabouts and switchbacks, the pleasures of vertigo, giddiness and some degree of anxiety. These pleasures too cannot be explained in terms of early oral experiences. He believes that the fundamental elements of all thrills consist of

(a) some amount of conscious fear, or at least an awareness of real external danger; (b) a voluntary and intentional exposing of oneself to this external danger and to the fear aroused by it; (c) while having the confident hope that the fear can be tolerated and mastered, the danger will pass, and that one will be able to return unharmed to safety.

(1959a: 23)

In order to be able to discuss the psychology of thrills, he followed his own advice and coined two new technical terms. To describe a person who enjoys thrills, he suggests the term 'philobat' and the abstract phenomenon, 'philobatism'. To describe the opposite of the philobat, a person who cannot stand swings and roundabouts but prefers to cling to something firm when his security is in danger, he suggests the term 'ocnophil', with the

abstract phenomenon, 'ocnophilia'. As I mentioned earlier in the Introduction, he did not do himself justice with these terms, because of their
harsh and awkward sound, and this may play some part in the fact that these
terms, while expressing important non-verbal concepts, have not caught
on with most readers.

These two primitive forms of object relationships are hardly ever
encountered in pure form and are usually found in varying mixtures, but
to start off with, one needs to examine the extreme forms.

> The ocnophilic world consists of objects, separated by horrid empty
> spaces. The ocnophil lives from object to object, cutting his sojourns
> in the empty spaces as short as possible. Fear is provoked by leaving
> the objects, and allayed by rejoining them . . . If the need is felt, the
> object must needs be there; moreover, in the state of need, no regard,
> consideration, or concern can be paid to the object, it is simply taken
> for granted. In other words, this means that the relation to an
> ocnophilic object is definitely predepressive.
>
> (1959a: 32–3)

Balint suggests that this type of object relationship is the best studied one
in psychoanalysis. At the other extreme,

> the philobatic world consists of friendly expanses dotted more or less
> densely with dangerous and unpredictable objects. One lives in the
> friendly expanses, carefully avoiding hazardous contacts with poten-
> tially dangerous objects. Whereas the ocnophilic world is structured
> by close proximity and touch, the philobatic world is structured by
> safe distance and sight.
>
> (1959a: 34)

The ocnophil lives in the illusion that his objects will protect him, whereas
the philobat's illusion is that his ego skills will protect him from hazardous,
potentially unfriendly objects. Thus the ocnophil has the compulsive need
to touch and be close to his object, whereas the philobat has the compulsive need to watch his environment for the potential emergence of
hazardous objects, upon which he will need to use his ego skills to convert
it into a friendly, or less dangerous, object. Balint includes among the ego
skills the emotional attitudes of regard, consideration, concern and looking
after, and therefore regards the philobatic attitude as being post-depressive
in origin (1959a: 36). However, he does cast doubt on this when he also
remarks that

> he is never in doubt that he can find new objects, new ideas, and he
> even enjoys dropping the old and finding the new. In a way it is only
> his freedom that matters, and seemingly he does not care much

whether he is loved or not, as he is certain that if need be he can make any object love him.

(1959a: 40)

This does not sound like an attitude of consideration, concern or looking after of the object but rather a pre-depressive part-object attitude of lack of concern and taking the object for granted and the projection of badness into the object.

Balint extends the ocnophilic and philobatic attitudes to include not only the world of external relationships with people but also the internal world of ideas and ideals. The ocnophil will cling strongly to his familiar world of ideas, beliefs and conventions and find it difficult to depart from them. The philobat, on the other hand, will enjoy dropping old ideas and will readily find new ones, but these will be no longer-lasting than those discarded. Such attitudes are of importance when one considers the problems of psychic change that need to occur in therapy.

He also examines these states in relation to aggressivity and auto-erotism, to love and hate, and to reality-testing. He concludes this first section on thrills with the view

that the philobat's confidence in his ability to cope with external dangers, in the friendliness of the expanses, and in his safe home-coming, was exaggerated and somewhat unrealistic, and in the same way the ocnophil's belief that his objects were safe, powerful and kind, was equally out of the true. We asked . . . what the mechanisms are enabling them to stick to their convictions in spite of the ubiquitous testimony of their experience, that other people have the extreme opposite view and events do not justify either of them. The search for the answers to these questions has led us to the assumption of a more primitive picture of the world which must be chronologically earlier than either the ocnophilic or the philobatic worlds. With this, how-ever, we must leave the common conventional world of adults and enter the primitive world of early infancy and of regression.

(1959a: 56)

In entering this world of early infancy and of regression in the second half of the book, Balint first conducts an extensive investigation into the etymology of the words 'object', 'subject' and 'matter'. These terms he relates to a study of the physiological psychology of the primitive senses, and he concludes that at one time

there must have been a harmonious mix-up in our minds between ourselves and the world around us, and that our 'mother' was involved in it. Though this mix-up strikes us as childish and primitive, we must admit that it preceded our 'modern', 'adult', or 'scientific'

picture of the world which, so to speak, grew out of it, and unde-
niably some of its primitive features were carried over into its later
form.

(1959a: 62)

He points out that the mixing-up of external and internal worlds is well
known in psychoanalysis, by virtue of the clinical phenomena of illusion
and hallucination, confusion, fugues, depersonalization, toxic states caused
by drugs, and the dynamic processes of projection and introjection. From
the study of regression in the analytic situation, we derive the phantasy of
'a primal harmony which by right ought to be our due and which was
destroyed either through our own fault, through the machinations of
others, or by our own cruel fate' (1959a: 64). This harmony is the theme
of a number of religious beliefs and fairy tales, and the experience may be
approached in sexual orgasm and in ecstasies. This harmonious state
accords with his theory of primary object-love, and from this state, the
presence of discrete, separate objects gradually emerges in the interaction
between the individual and his environment. The traumatic discovery of
their existence must be accepted, and as a secondary result of this, there
arise the two basic attitudes of philobatism and ocnophilia by which the
individual responds to this discovery, with many gradations and shades
between them.

Balint believes that 'the two most important senses that provide the
perceptions which form the basis for the discovery of "objects" are sight
and touch. Both are undeveloped in the first post-natal months, as they
both need a considerable degree of muscular coordination to work
properly' (1959a: 62). (This view does not accord with the newest research
on mother–infant interaction, which suggests that the visual awareness of
the environment is present from birth.) If this is factually the case, the
harmonious mix-up would not occur as a post-natal state, but would
represent a pre-natal state, one experienced in the womb. Balint, in fact,
mentions this possibility in passing when he is discussing the chronology of
ocnophilia and philobatism (1959a: 84).

He now turns to the discussion of regression in the analytic situation.

In quite a number of my analyses, there occurs a period in which the
patient feels a very strong urge or need to get up from the couch.
Some patients are content to sit up, others want to stand – more often
than not in a safe corner of the room farthest from my chair – and yet
others have to walk about. Obviously this 'acting-out' is overdetermined. . . . There is also the fact that it takes the patient away
from a hazardous object, his analyst, and opens up for him expanses,
which, though not entirely friendly, are still felt to be less dangerous
or less exciting than the proximity of the analyst. . . . It is fair to say

that in many respects these episodes are reminiscent of the philobatic states we have described . . . if correctly recognized and handled by the analyst, [it] reveals itself almost always as an important experience, a piece of working through, leading towards a better mutual understanding between patient and analyst. The establishment of this better understanding mainly depends upon whether or not the analyst can achieve a change in the patient's fantasy from a hazardous object into part of the friendly expanses which need no longer be defied or watched with suspicion.

(1959a: 93)

With other patients,

a number of them start analysis with their eyes open, interested in and intent, almost anxiously, watching the objects around them in the consulting room. It is only very gradually that they discover the possibility of closing their eyes, detaching their ocnophilic clinging attention from the objects of the external world, and turning to the events in their own minds. . . . It is only after long and intensive work on this second level that they can open their eyes and look round in the world which is then no longer hostile.

(1959a: 93)

These and similar phenomena are recognized as overdetermined in origin, with ocnophilic and philobatic tendencies being two of the determinants. He now adds a view that denotes a change from his earlier one on these regressive states.

I thought that the need to be near to the analyst, to touch or to cling to him, was one of the most characteristic features of primary love. Now I realize that the need to cling is a reaction to a trauma, an expression of, and a defence against, the fear of being dropped or abandoned. It is therefore a secondary phenomenon only, its aim being the restoration by proximity and touch of the original, subject-object identity . . . what I call primary object relation or primary love.

(1959a: 100)

This change of view concerning touching and clinging is of great importance since it concerns one of the controversial issues of technique in regressive states. The issue is whether there should be any physical touching or holding between patient and analyst. We shall return to this issue when it is discussed in the next chapter, on *The Basic Fault*.

Finally, Balint discusses what he calls the ocnophilic and philobatic bias of our theory and technique. With patients who tend to go into a regressed state, some analysts will regard such regressions with suspicion, calling it acting-out, and interpreting any move towards them as the patient's attempt to escape from the analytic work. Other analysts may tolerate regressions but nevertheless force the patients out of them by their otherwise correct interpretations, since the acceptance and the understanding of interpretations demands more maturity from the patient than the state of regression can afford. Balint believes that these techniques, and particularly the interpretation of everything in the analytic situation primarily as transference, means that the analyst offers himself incessantly as an object to his patient, almost demands to be clung to, and consistently interprets anything contrary to clinging as an attempt to escape from the analytic work. This results in 'a highly ocnophilic theory of object relationships founded primarily on part-objects, and . . . we have made great advances in developing a theory of frustration and of ambivalence' (1959a: 102). Balint's criticism of Fairbairn's theoretical position described in the previous chapter was precisely on this issue. This may well lead to the patient being induced to introject an idealized image of his analyst, in exchanging one set of ocnophilic internal objects for another, which, although it may be helpful therapeutically since the new set is better adapted to reality, may also not be helpful in enabling the patient to stand on his own feet and see with his own eyes, as Balint puts it.

He does nevertheless notice that despite this concept of the present ocnophilic technique, the published accounts of patients' imagery in describing their subjective experiences at the end of their treatment shows them to be philobatic in nature, with phrases such as 'the world has opened up for him', 'as long as he can stand on his own feet', 'his eyes are now sweeping new horizons'. This makes him feel that his criticism of present technique may be 'unjust and incomplete, inasmuch as there must be other strong forces at work' (1959a: 105). He does not, however, suggest what these other forces may be, but I would myself postulate that one of these forces may be contained in the very nature and structure of a transference interpretation. In such an interpretation, there is always an expressing of the patient–analyst relationship in the immediacy of the here-and-now, and hence an implied separation verbally expressed by the use of the words 'you' and 'me', a separation of subject and object. Consistency in interpreting and expressing this verbal separation will have the effect of gradually allowing the patient to experience this separation, and in this way, to facilitate the process of his standing on his own feet and seeing with his own eyes.

The philobatic technique, according to Balint, also has its problems. This technique would use easily understandable interpretations very sparingly, and the analyst would simply remain alive and available to the patient in his regressions. The danger is that it may well leave too much to the patient, forcing on him too much independence too early, and so lead to the introjection of a demanding figure exacting heroic standards from his poor patients.

This leads Balint to offer both a structural and a dynamic theory to account for his two character types.

> The result of this kind of introjection – no matter whether it was forced upon the patient by ocnophilic or philobatic techniques – is the acquisition of an efficient shell. This shell has a double function. It supplies the individual with various skills necessary for life, but at the same time it restricts his possibilities of experiencing either love or hatred, either joy or misery. Life will reach him only with such intensity and in such form as his shell allows. One gets the impression that the ocnophil's objects are in a way part of his shell, hence his highly ambivalent feelings towards them. On the other hand, the philobat's adventures while courting real dangers in search of thrills may be rebellious attempts to crack by realistic fears the efficient shell in order to get in touch with his real self hidden behind it. Neither of these states allows much freedom to feel or indeed to live; their development should be watched and avoided, in education as well as during analytic treatment.
>
> (1959a: 107)

The book now ends, but in an Appendix, entitled 'Distance in Space and Time', Enid Balint extends his concepts to cover the influence of distances, not just in space but also in time:

> It could be said that philobats are people who have overcome at an early age the difficulty caused by the time-lag between one satisfaction and the next by transferring their enjoyment and love from the satisfactory moment itself to their ability to pass through the time between two satisfactions. The ocnophils, never having overcome the difficulty of the time between satisfactions, have come either to deny its existence or to flee from anything that is reminiscent of the early difficulty.
>
> (1959a: 127)

She concludes, 'The ocnophil avoids the distances between objects and satisfactions and tries to deny their existence; the philobat transfers parts of his libido from direct satisfaction to a skilful overcoming of the unsatisfactory spaces and times between satisfactions' (1959a: 131).

I have found these concepts of ocnophilia and philobatism useful in clinical practice in thinking about the technique of interpretation. As Balint describes it, if one interprets too much of the immediate here-and-now of the transference–counter-transference, the danger is the development of an ocnophilic clinging to the analyst, which may encourage an interminable analysis. On the other hand, too little interpretation of this aspect may encourage acting-out and a premature pseudo-maturity in the patient of a philobatic type. The optimum is often not easy to ascertain. Other than this consideration of interpretation, I would expect that Balint's ideas will become far more relevant in psychoanalytic thinking when the influence of the non-verbal, sensual, bodily aspects of the analytic relationship come into focus in our clinical theories.

4

The Basic Fault (1968)

We now come to Balint's last book, which gathers together much of his thinking on theoretical and technical concepts as they have been described previously. In addition, however, he is still extending his thoughts and adding further concepts, even suggesting at the end of the book future pathways by which the work could be extended. It is important to note that the subtitle of the book is 'Therapeutic Aspects of Regression', since it is in this area that the greatest advances are described.

In the first part of the book he introduces the concept of the three areas of the mind: the area of the Oedipal level, the area of the basic fault and the area of creation. He starts by wondering why some patients who have been judged suitable for analytic treatment are more difficult to treat than others, and why some analyses are less rewarding to analyst and patient than others. He suggests that we do not have a great deal of knowledge of the therapeutic processes and of the changes that may occur in the id, ego and superego in these processes. He also suggests that we have even less knowledge of the relationship between these processes and changes and the different techniques that are used by analysts of different schools, and that possibly the different schools succeed or fail with different sorts of patients. He notes how any research into this topic seems to arouse great anxiety and resistance among analysts.

He then discusses one aspect of interpretation, in that an interpretation consists of sentences made up of words which have an agreed meaning to both analyst and patient. If the ego is sufficiently strong, the interpretation is 'taken in' by the patient and followed by 'working-through' as described by Freud. Problems will arise when interpretations are not taken in as such, and normal working-through cannot then occur.

From this, Balint conceptualized two levels of analytic work occurring in two areas of the mind, which he described as the Oedipal level and the level of the basic fault. The most important difference between them concerns language. At the Oedipal level, the patient can 'take in' interpretations, as words mean the same to both analyst and patient, and 'working-through' can occur. These interpretations may be of pre-Oedipal, pre-genital as well as Oedipal material, but they are still verbally at the Oedipal level. At the other level, the level of the basic fault, this taking-in of the interpretation does not occur, as adult, or agreed, or conventional language is often misleading or useless to the patient since words no longer have their agreed or conventional meaning.

> This important difference with regard to language, which may create a gulf between patient and analyst and obstruct the progress of treatment, was first described by Ferenczi, in particular in his last Congress paper (1932) and in his posthumously published 'Notes and Fragments'. He called it 'The Confusion of Tongues between the Child [singular!] and the Adults [plural!]'.
>
> (1968: 15)

The other difference between these two levels is that at the Oedipal level, everything happens in a relationship consisting of three or more persons, and the problems encountered are always associated with conflict; at the basic fault level, all events belong to a two-person relationship and the dynamic force operating in the mind is not one of conflict but of a fault. This word is used in its geological sense, and not the moral, and describes a sudden irregularity in the overall structure which under stress may lead to a break, which profoundly disrupts this overall structure. In the mind, the form of the fault is of the experience of something distorted or lacking in the mind which produces a defect that must be put right. In addition, there is a feeling that the cause of this fault is that someone has either failed or defaulted on the patient; together with this, there is great anxiety that the analyst should not fail the patient.

Having defined this level, he now describes the clinical signs in the analysis that would indicate that the basic fault level has been reached. These are

1 a profound change in the atmosphere of the analysis from the previously fairly conventional smoothness and understanding state;
2 that interpretations are now experienced as persecutory or seductive statements;
3 that ordinary words tend to lose their conventional meanings and every gesture or movement of the analyst assumes great importance;
4 the patient seems able to get under the analyst's skin and understand the analyst's behaviour with great accuracy, except that it is lopsided and out of proportion;
5 the patient may show parapsychological phenomena such as telepathy or clairvoyance;

6 if the analyst fails to respond to the patient as the patient expects him to, the reaction is not of anger or criticism but of feelings of emptiness, deadness and futility, with an apparently lifeless acceptance of everything offered by the analyst; or perhaps persecutory anxieties may arise of the analyst being deliberately malicious or malevolent towards the patient;

7 in spite of this, the patient shows great determination to get on with things in the analysis.

Although Balint does not call it such, these indications of the clinical state seem to suggest a borderline transference psychosis. Balint's originality in his description of this state is shown by the inclusion of parapsychological phenomena, which would certainly have been appreciated by Freud and Ferenczi with their well-known interest in this 'non-respectable' scientific area of research.

I also think that, although Balint does not explicitly describe it as such, the sense of his writing may convey that the language of the basic fault is that of a child, as compared with the adult language of the Oedipal level. His citing of the 'Confusion of Tongues', which concerns adults and children, may add weight to this. He gives no clinical example of what he actually means, but I would suggest from my own clinical experience of such patients that he is not speaking of the language of normal children but rather the pathological language of primitive concrete symbolism which has resulted from the partial breakdown of the normal adult symbolic language at the Oedipal level. Words tend to lose their socially accepted overtones of understanding together with their clusters of associations.

The origins of the basic fault may be traced back to the early formative years of the individuals when there was a discrepancy between their bio-psychological needs and the material and psychological care, attention and affection available to them. To repeat the earlier description in 'The Doctor, His Patient and the Illness':

> this creates a state of deficiency whose consequences and after-effects appear to be only partly reversible. The cause of this early discrepancy may be congenital, i.e. the infant's bio-psychological needs may have been too exacting (there are non-viable infants and progressive congenital conditions, like Friedreich's ataxia or cystic kidneys), or may be environmental, such as care that is insufficient, deficient, haphazard, over-anxious, over-protective, harsh, rigid, grossly inconsistent, incorrectly timed, over-stimulating, or merely un-understanding or indifferent.

He emphasizes the lack of 'fit' between the child and the people representing its environment and notes the similarity to the lack of 'fit' earlier

49

observed between the analyst's correct technique and a particular patient's needs. He believes this to be an important cause of the difficulties and failures experienced by analysts in their clinical practice.

The third area of the mind, according to Balint, is what he calls the area of creation, in which belong artistic creation, science and mathematics, philosophy, the gaining of insight and, interestingly, the early phases of becoming mentally and physically ill, and the spontaneous recovery from such an illness. This area is of a one-person relationship, where there is no external object and hence no external object relationship and no transference. This results in there being nothing very clear for the analyst to explore, which makes any knowledge of the processes involved scanty and uncertain.

He suggests that even though the subject is on his own, 'somethings' are there in this area of the mind and he proposes the term 'pre-object', to cover this something. He thinks that Bion (1962, 1963) had similar problems in conceptualizing these processes for which he had suggested the use of the terms 'alpha- and beta-elements', and 'alpha-functioning'. The pre-objects are primitive, not organized or whole, and only after the work of creation do they become organized, whole and capable of a proper verbal description and definition. He suggests that the only thing known of this process of creation is that it is unpredictable in its success or failure, and that the speed of creation can vary from very slow to lightning fast. He further suggests that conflicts at the Oedipal level could accelerate or inhibit the speed of the process, but in the final resort, it is the structure of the area of creation that really matters.

To recapitulate, Balint describes three areas of the mind: the area of creation, the area of the basic fault, and the area of the Oedipal level. Each area is characterized by the presence of one, two and three or more external objects, a psychology first proposed by John Rickman (1951). Each area has its own particular characteristics which have been set out above, and from here, we can now proceed to his discussion of two of the theories that have for long been at the centre of Balint's thinking, those of primary narcissism and primary object-love.

Since 1935 ('Critical Notes on the Theory of the Pre-genital Organizations of the Libido'), he had insisted that narcissism is always a secondary phenomenon and never primary, and in the second section of *The Basic Fault* (1968), he gives his most extensive critique of primary narcissism. He notes that Freud, at different times, had proposed three theories about the individual's most primitive relationship with his environment. These three theories are primary object relationship, primary auto-erotism and primary narcissism, and although they contradict one another, this contradiction was never discussed by Freud. Rather, Freud attempted a synthesis of these theories in favour of primary narcissism, yet this new synthesis itself now contained inherent contradictions. Balint also notes that the clinical observations that had been used by Freud and then others to justify the acceptance of this theory in fact only demonstrate the existence of secondary narcissism. The observations cited include the study of schizophrenia and psychosis, homosexuality, organic diseases, hypochondriasis, the erotic life of the sexes, various overvaluations of self and others, sleep, and observations of infants and young children. Balint then proposes that his own theory of primary object-love, which is recapitulated in this section, makes these phenomena better understandable and more integrated with one another than the primary narcissism theory.

In his chapter on 'Primary Love', Balint gives his most complete account of his theory of the early development of object relations. Since he has described the earliest state of primary object-love in libidinal terms, he has cast this account of development in terms of the libidinal cathexis of objects:

> According to my theory, the individual is born in a state of intense relatedness to his environment, both biologically and libidinally. Prior to birth, self and environment are harmoniously 'mixed up', in fact, they interpenetrate each other. In this world, as has been mentioned, there are as yet no objects, only limitless substances or expanses.
>
> Birth is a trauma that upsets this equilibrium by changing the environment radically and enforces – under a real threat of death – a new form of adaptation. This starts off or, at any rate considerably accelerates, the separation between individual and environment. Objects, including the ego, begin to emerge from the mix-up of substances and from the breaking up of the harmony of the limitless expanses. The objects have – in contrast to the friendlier substances – firm contours and sharp boundaries which henceforth must be recognized and respected. Libido is no longer in a homogeneous flux from the id to the environment; under the influence of the emerging objects, concentrations and rarefactions appear in its flow.
>
> Wherever the developing relationship to a part of the environment or to an object is in painful contrast to the earlier undisturbed harmony, libido may be withdrawn to the ego, which starts or accelerates developing – perhaps as a consequence of the enforced new adaptation – in an attempt to regain the previous feeling of 'oneness' of the first stages. This part of the libido would be definitely narcissistic, but secondary to the original environment cathexis. Accordingly the libidinal cathexes observed in early infancy would be of four sorts:
>
> (a) remnants of the original environment cathexis transferred to the emerging objects,

(b) other remnants of the original environment cathexis withdrawn
to the ego as secondary comforters against frustration, i.e. narcissistic and auto-erotic cathexes, and

(c) re-cathexes emanating from the secondary narcissism of the ego.
In addition to these three fairly well-studied forms of cathexis
there is a fourth which results in

(d) the development of the ocnophilic and the philobatic structures
of the world.

(1968: 67–8)

Balint does not elaborate in item (c) on what he means by 're-cathexes
emanating from the secondary narcissism of the ego' except to say that it is
a fairly well-studied form of cathexis. I would suggest that he is probably
referring to Klein's paranoid and depressive stages of development, since in
his 1952 paper he considers them to be secondary narcissistic states developing from the earlier stage of primary love.

Parts 3, 4 and 5 are concerned with the techniques and problems that
arise in the analysis of regressed patients. Part 3 is concerned with the
important problem of communicating with a patient regressed to the level
of the basic fault, where conventional adult language is no longer understood as such by the patient. He describes this as the task of 'bridging the
gulf' separating the adult analyst from the 'child in the patient'. In the area
of the basic fault, the patient's non-verbal communications are equal in
importance to his verbal utterances, whether one calls them 'behaviour',
'repetition', 'acting-out', and so on, and one of the analyst's tasks is to
'translate' for the patient his primitive, non-verbal behaviour by acting not
only as an 'interpreter' but also as an 'informer' – that is, by helping the
patient to become aware of what he has been doing in the analytic
situation.

In order to perform this task, the analyst must use language – in this
instance an analytic language – and the nature and form of this language
will vary from analyst to analyst, depending on their different theoretical
and technical assumptions on the fundamentals of psychoanalysis. These
languages will be heavily based on the type of language used by the
analyst's analyst and supervisors, and from this Balint proceeds to discuss
briefly three of these languages, which are very roughly equivalent to those
belonging to the three groups of the British Psycho-Analytical Society.

The classical technique was the language used by Freud to describe both
Oedipal and pre-Oedipal experiences, which means for Balint that they are
interpreted in adult language. Most of the phenomena belonging to the
basic fault will tend to be attributed to castration anxiety or penis envy,
which are two of the overdetermining factors. This can be therapeutically
effective, but if this is not the case, then the patients are considered to have

been unsuitable for psychoanalysis and the fault for this would be held to lie in the selection criteria of patients for treatment. If the parameters of technique, such as frequency of sessions, duration of sessions, abstinence and so forth are altered, there remains the danger of their becoming irreversible.

The Klein group has a language and technique of interpretation of its own, particularly for the description of experiences at the primitive levels. One aspect of this is that the patient relates at a part-object level, and use is made of nouns like 'milk', 'breast', 'contents inside the body', and so on, and verbs like 'split off', 'take in', 'project', 'persecute', 'damage', and so on. Patients are reported as experiencing this language as something mad being forced onto them, yet consistent use of this language may be therapeutically helpful to the patient. The limitations appear to be of introjection and idealization of the analyst and his technique, and a reluctance to admit therapeutic failure. It is interesting to note that since this critique of Balint's was published, the use of this part-object language has been replaced by a more gradual approach to bodily expressions of unconscious phantasy (Spillius 1983), but this may not necessarily be an instance of cause and effect.

The third group, who are mainly those who have been influenced by Ferenczi (1932) and Winnicott's ideas (1954) on regression, deal with the phenomena encountered at the level of the basic fault by means of management in addition to understanding and interpretation. By the term 'management' is meant nursing, protecting, mediating, looking after, physical holding and so on as the patient regresses to the state of dependence on the analyst. Very briefly, the theory behind this is that a suitable atmosphere must be created in which interpretations can reach and become intelligible to the real self of the patient, which up till then has been hidden behind the patient's false self ('Metapsychological and Clinical Aspects of Regression within the Psychoanalytical Set-up', Winnicott 1954). This can occasionally be therapeutically effective but more often, after some initial improvement, the patient develops a spiralling of needs and demands on the analyst, which eventually results in a breakdown of the analysis. It is in the further understanding of the phenomena and problems that are created by this form of management that Balint's theoretical and technical position has become so important.

This position is developed in the next section of the book, entitled 'The Benign and the Malignant Forms of Regression'. He starts by discussing Freud's historical usage of the term 'regression', and shows that clinically it describes four functions. These are (1) as a mechanism of defence, (2) as a factor in pathogenesis, (3) as a potent form of transference resistance, and (4) as an essential factor in analytic therapy. Freud had distinguished three aspects of regression, the topographic, the temporal and the formal, and it is formal regression that is of importance in therapeutic regression. From his experience with regressed patients, Freud had become very wary of dealing with them in any way other than by interpretation and by maintaining an atmosphere of privation and abstinence in not gratifying his patient's needs and demands. Ferenczi, however, had continued to experiment by offering gratifications since he had experienced occasional therapeutic success and he was impressed by patients' responses to him. He believed that the pathogenesis of mental illness lay in traumatic behaviours by adults when the patient was an infant, which was not acknowledged as such by the adult. He thought that the analytic situation re-created the needs and demands of the past towards the analyst, who remains in a state of objective, sympathetic detachment towards his patient, and thereby re-creates by this attitude the original traumatic situation. He then tried numerous techniques, including mutual analysis, as described in his *Clinical Diary* (1988), to prevent this happening by trying '(a) to help the patient to regress to the traumatic situation, (b) to watch carefully what degree of tension the patient will be able to bear in this state, and (c) to see to it that the tension will remain at about that level by responding positively to the regressed patient's longings, cravings or needs' (1968: 126). Balint remarks here that this therapeutic research was the first intensive study of the doctor–patient relationship and led to the discovery of the technique of counter-transference interpretations.

However, when physical holding and kissing were introduced into these experimental techniques, Freud felt obliged to admonish Ferenczi, leading to the rift that developed between them. Freud predicted that 'it would prove impossible to satisfy unconditionally every need of a regressed patient, that any attempt of this kind would improve the patient's state only as long as the analyst was able and willing to be at the patient's beck and call and, lastly, that most of these patients, even though improved, would never become really independent' (1968: 126).

Balint now discusses his own experiences in this field and describes the case of a young female patient who, in the second year of her analysis, was enabled during a session to perform a somersault for the first time in her life. This was the prelude to many further changes in her personal, social and professional life, all of which proved to be long-lasting in their effects. He comments that such behaviour could be conceptualized as basic fault, acting-out, repetition and regression, although none of these concepts fits in completely with the performance of this somersault. Accordingly, he uses the term 'regression' 'to denote rather loosely the emergence in response to analytic treatment of primitive forms of behaving and experiencing, after more mature forms have firmly established themselves' (1968: 129). Regression, defined in this way, is then differentiated from other clinical states which resemble regression, such as withdrawal from the analyst or the environment, absorption in one's area of creation and states of disintegration.

However, Balint also recognizes that

> one could argue that the decisive factor in bringing about the good therapeutic result was the analytic work that preceded the incident described [the somersault], and the proper working-through that followed it. The incident itself, though impressive, was insignificant, apart perhaps from permitting some harmless relief from the strenuous work both to the patient and her analyst. It is difficult to answer this argument on the basis of a successful case.

He describes further examples of patients where certain forms of gratification were accepted as appropriate by the analyst. These include such gratifications as the allowing of extra sessions; the analyst telephoning the patient at the weekend at a certain stage in the analysis; allowing the patient to be silent; the allowing of the patient to hold the analyst's finger. Following these gratifications, he reports that the patient's relationships change in that it 'opened up new ways of loving and hating for the patient. This amounted to a new discovery, and from then on the patient's relationship towards her objects of love and hate became freer and more realistic' (1968: 131). These experiences, 'new beginnings', are characterized by a particular analytic atmosphere, which he called '*arglos*', a German adjective approximately meaning innocent, guileless, harmless, and it is important that it is only in such an atmosphere that such gratifications are permitted.

He thought that this *arglos* atmosphere and the new beginning experiences would resemble that of the primary object-love relationship; that there is a phase prior to the appearance of primary objects which, he says,

> might be called the phase of the undifferentiated environment, the phase of the primary substances, or – a somewhat clumsy phrase – the phase of the harmonious interpenetrating mix-up . . . the best illustration for this state is the relationship we have towards the air surrounding us. It is difficult to say whether the air in our lungs or in our guts is us, or not us; and it does not even matter . . . as long as it is there, the relationship between us and it cannot be observed, or only with great difficulty; if, however, anything interferes with our supply of air, impressive and noisy symptoms develop in the same way as with the dissatisfied infant, or with the unsatisfied patient in the first phase of the new beginning.
>
> (1968: 136)

By the term 'primary substances', Balint means the ancient philosophical elements of water, earth, fire and air. Their chief characteristic is their indestructibility, and Balint maintains that the analyst's role in certain periods of new beginning resembles this. 'He must be there; he must be pliable to a very high degree; he must not offer much resistance; he certainly must be indestructible, and he must allow his patients to live with him in a sort of harmonious interpenetrating mix-up' (1968: 136). He does not enlarge on this with any clinical examples, but I believe that by the last part he means that one should not try by interpretative means to undo any projective and introjective identifications that may be present in this transference situation in which there is a relative de-differentiation between subject and object. He did, however, emphasize strongly that experiencing gratification does not replace interpretation but is in addition to it. The crucial aspect is that the interpretation is made after the patient has the experience, not during it, since otherwise the experience of the gratification and what it may symbolize will be destroyed by the patient being asked to focus on the interpretation.

He also noted that several other analysts had described this sort of relationship of being like an indestructible primary substance in their own particular terms: 'need-satisfying object' (A. Freud), 'average expectable environment' (Hartmann), 'container and contained' (Bion), 'holding function of mother' (Winnicott), and so on.

This, as Balint says, is the positive side of the situation, but unfortunately there are negative sides too. In his clinical experience,

> patients fall into two groups: in some treatments only one, or at most a few, periods of regression or new beginning occurred, after which the patient spontaneously emerged from his primitive world and felt better, or was even cured – as predicted by Ferenczi: while with some others it seemed that they could never have enough; as soon as one of their primitive wishes or needs was satisfied, it was replaced by a new wish or craving, equally demanding and urgent. This in some cases led to the development of addiction-like states which were difficult to handle, and in some cases proved – as Freud predicted – intractable.
>
> (1968: 138)

He suggests that in the first group, the patient in his regression expects the tacit consent of the analyst to use the external world in a way that would allow him to get on with his internal problems, to be able to reach himself. In the second group, the regression is aimed at a gratification of his instinctual cravings by an action of the external world, his analyst. He calls the first type 'regression aimed at recognition', and the second 'regression aimed at gratification'. The first type he also refers to as 'benign regression', and the second 'malignant regression'. He now proceeds to set out the clinical features of these two types:

Most cases belonging to the benign form of regression show:

1 not much difficulty in establishing a mutually trusting *arglos* unsuspecting relationship, which is reminiscent of the primary relationship towards primary substances;
2 a regression, leading to a true new beginning, in particular of the patient's internal problems;
3 the regression is for the sake of recognition, in particular, of the patient's internal problems;
4 only moderately high intensity of the demands, expectations or 'needs';
5 absence of signs of severe hysteria in the clinical symptomatology and of genital-orgastic elements in the regressed transference.

In contrast, most cases belonging to the malignant form of regression show the following picture:

1 since the mutually trusting relationship is highly precariously balanced, the *arglos*, unsuspecting, atmosphere breaks down repeatedly, and frequently symptoms of desperate clinging develop as safeguards and reassurance against another possible breakdown;
2 a malignant form of regression, several unsuccessful attempts at reaching a new beginning, a constant threat of unending spiral of demands or needs, and of development of addiction-like states;
3 the regression is aimed at gratification by external action;
4 suspiciously high intensity of demands, expectations, or 'needs';
5 presence of signs of severe hysteria in the clinical picture and of genital-orgastic elements both in the normal and in the regressed form of transference.

(1968: 146)

He remarks that in most cases of therapeutic regression, the analyst sees a mixture of these features but usually one type prevails; he adds that in his experience, malignant regression occurs in patients suffering from hysteria or hysterical character disorder.

The differentiation of these two types of regression would essentially rest on three criteria. The first is that malignant regression usually occurs in the earlier phases of the analysis whereas benign regression tends to occur in the later phases. The second is that in malignant regression, gratification is demanded of something from the analyst, whereas in benign regression, the demand is usually for the analyst to be there. The third is that in malignant regression, the atmosphere or mood as experienced in the countertransference is usually intense and passionate, whereas in the benign regression it is calmer and trusting. However, this is not always the case and the issue of the atmosphere is discussed in a later chapter on further developments.

Balint now emphasizes that the form the regression will take, whether it be benign or malignant, depends not only on the patient, his personality and his illness, but also on the way he is responded to by his object, the analyst. This means that regression is not simply an intrapsychic phenomenon but also an intersubjective and interpersonal one, and Balint now considers the response of the analyst to his regressed patient.

He reminds us that, in his view, if the patient's compulsive patterns and object relationships originate from conflicts and complexes within the patient, appropriate interpretations can help the patient to resolve them. If, however, the compulsive patterns originate in a reaction to the basic fault, interpretations will have incomparably less power as (1) there is not a conflict or complex to be solved by interpretation, and (2) words in the area of the basic fault have lost most of their reliability as therapeutic tools. He believes that in these cases additional therapeutic agents, besides interpretations, must be considered, and that

> the most important of these is to help the patient to develop a primitive relationship in the analytic situation corresponding to his compulsive pattern and maintain it in undisturbed peace till he can discover the possibility of new forms of object relationship, experience them, and experiment with them . . . a necessary task if the treatment is to inactivate the basic fault by creating conditions in which it can head off.
>
> (1968: 166)

In order to foster this development, he suggested three important things that the analyst should avoid doing. The first is to avoid interpreting everything first as transference, since he believes that this 'tempts us to turn into mighty and knowledgeable objects for our patients, thus helping – or forcing – them to regress into an ocnophilic world' (1968: 166). The second is 'not to become, or to behave, as a separate sharply-contoured object . . . [but to] allow his patients to relate to, or exist with, him as if he were one of the primary substances' (1968: 167). Balint seems to be implying in this that the analyst should tolerate some forms of acting-out and should also accept the patient's projective and introjective identifications without wanting to hurry to interpret them back to the patient. The third thing is to avoid becoming or appearing omnipotent.

> This is one of the most difficult tasks in this period of the treatment. The regressed patient expects his analyst to know more, and to be more powerful; if nothing else, the analyst is expected to promise, either explicitly or by his behaviour, that he will help his patient out of the regression, or see the patient through it. Any such promise, even the slightest appearance of a tacit agreement towards it, will

create very great difficulties, almost insurmountable obstacles, for the analytic work.

(1968: 167)

He describes the analyst in this phase of his work as the 'unobtrusive analyst'; this is a far cry from the techniques used by Ferenczi in his attempts to reach his regressed patients. These had included active techniques, whereby the analyst had either forbidden the patient from performing certain actions in order to increase the tension between patient and analyst, or had encouraged the patient to relax in order to lessen the tension. These being unsuccessful, he had spoken of his counter-transference feelings to the patients themselves. This had helped temporarily but not for long, and the next experiment was of 'mutual analysis', whereby the analyst and patient took turns at 'analysing' each other. This was sometimes accompanied by physical contact and kissing. Ferenczi had eventually realized that none of these procedures had been really helpful in many cases, but his death in 1933 brought an end to further experiments (Ferenczi, *Clinical Diary*, 1988). Balint had eschewed all these techniques, advocating the stance of the unobtrusive analyst, but he still occasionally allowed finger-holding, when he judged the atmosphere to be appropriately *arglos*; this seems to be the final remnant of his positive attachment to this aspect of Ferenczi's technique. Perhaps Ferenczi had used it during Balint's analysis with him to Balint's benefit. Nevertheless, this advocacy of finger-holding, even if the atmosphere is judged to be correct, has been called into question by myself (Stewart, 'Technique at the Basic Fault: Regression', 1989) and will be discussed in Chapter 6, on 'Critiques and Further Developments'.

Balint constantly emphasizes that the acceptance of experiences of acting-out and regression without speedy interpretation, the use of the object relationship as the therapeutic agent, did not mean that interpretation was to be neglected. It meant that the interpretations for facilitating understanding and insight into the dynamics of the regression and the transference were to be given after the emergence from the regressed state. The non-verbal communication had to be experienced in its own right and intensity and, only later, be put into organized verbal utterances. He also made the point, however, that interpretations should be given 'if the analyst is certain that the patient needs them, for at such times not giving them would be felt as unwarranted demand or stimulation' (1968: 180).

He suggests that the allowing of the patient to regress into himself is connected with his ideas on the area of creation. In this area,

there is no external organized object, and any intrusion of such an object by attention-seeking interpretations inevitably destroys for the patient the possibility of creating something out of himself . . . objects

59

in this area are as yet unorganized, and the process of creation leading to their creation needs, above all, time. This time may be short or very long; but whatever its length, it cannot be influenced from outside. Almost certainly the same will be true about our patients' creations out of their unconscious. This may be one of the reasons why the analyst's usual interpretations are felt by patients regressed to this area as inadmissible; interpretations are indeed whole, 'organized', thoughts or objects whose interactions with the hazy, dreamlike, as yet 'unorganized' contents of the area of creation might cause either havoc or an unnatural, premature organization.

(1968: 176)

The book concludes with his indicating the directions to be taken for his future thinking, which he calls the missing chapters of this book. They include the function of repetition, of acting-out, in therapy; the potential ways open to a patient to change his internal world which largely determines his relationship to external objects; the technical means available to help achieve such a change; and the functions of interpretations. Regrettably, he did not live to write them.

To sum up, this book has taken us through the development of his thinking on his chosen topics of the development of object relations and of psychoanalytic technique. He has delineated his theory of the three areas of the mind in terms of one-, two- and three- or more person psychology and their different modes of functioning in relation to creation, deficiency and conflict. His critique of the concept of primary narcissism and his advocacy of the concept of primary object-love has been sharpened and strengthened following his earlier formulations. Differences in technique for dealing with regressed patients as exemplified by the three groups of the British Psycho-Analytical Society are courageously examined and evaluated for their therapeutic potential. This leads on to his extensive delineation of the concepts of benign and malignant regression and his advice and recommendations for the analyst's technique in dealing with these regressed states, giving rise to the concept of the unobtrusive analyst. By his own creative research and thinking, Balint has vindicated those of Ferenczi.

5

A theory of trauma and psychoanalytic education

A number of Balint's papers have not been incorporated into book form, and I select those on two topics that add originality of thought to psycho-analysis. The first topic is a theory of trauma and the second, observations on psychoanalytical education.

The paper, 'Trauma and Object Relationship', was written in 1969 for the last number of Volume 50 of the *International Journal of Psycho-Analysis* to celebrate the half-century of its publication. Balint first examines Freud's ideas on trauma, and he shows that

> psychoanalysis had two theories for the aetiology of the neuroses. The older one of the two assumes the existence of an early sexual trauma and our understanding of its effects is based essentially on metapsychological, i.e. economic, considerations. The crucial event comes from outside, and the individual is unprepared for it, it causes a break in the protective shield against stimuli and floods the mind with an excessive amount of excitation. In order to deal with the excessive amount of stimulation, a compulsion to repeat is set in motion, the clinical expression of which is in certain cases a neurotic symptom.
>
> The new [second] theory starts with the assumption that the trauma, in spite of its appearance, is not an external event; it is produced by the individual himself as a fantasy. It cannot claim easily that the individual was unprepared and was flooded by an excessive amount of excitation because, after all, it was he himself who produced the phantasy; on the other hand, it can claim the existence of very high intensity strains between the various parts of the mental apparatus, for instance, the id which forced the ego to indulge in fantasy-making and the super-ego which orders that this activity should be suppressed. . . . I propose to call this new theory essentially structural.
>
> (1969: 430)

He notes that in *Analysis Terminable and Interminable* (1937: 220), Freud suggested the term 'alteration of the ego', which is the result of an interaction between congenital factors and very early experiences, to cover this structural type of aetiology; this contains a notion of possible very early traumas, even in the structural theory.

Clinical experience makes it difficult for it to be decided whether trauma or traumas have taken place and this gave rise to the introduction of several concepts of qualified traumas, such as partial trauma, strain trauma, cumulative trauma, screen trauma and so on. Balint believes that the introduction of these qualified traumas has occurred because the theory is incomplete, and he suggests a new triphasic theory of traumas, which in essence resembles the views put forward by Ferenczi in his 'Confusion of Tongues' paper, which also concerns traumatogenesis in childhood.

> In the first phase the immature child is dependent on the adult and, although frustrations in their relationship may occur which may lead to irritation and even to rage at times, the relationship between the child and the adult is mainly trusting. In the second phase the adult, contrary to the child's expectation, does something highly exciting, frightening, or painful; this may happen once and quite suddenly or repeatedly . . . In any of these cases there exists for a time a most intense, often passionate, interacting between the child and the adult. It seems that this phase in itself, although it may appear to be very impressive, does not always act traumatically. The real completion of the trauma sets in in the third phase when the child, either having in mind the adult's passionate participation in the events of the second phase, approaches his partner again with a wish and an offer to continue the exciting, passionate game, or, still in pain and distress about the fact that in the previous phase his approach remained unrecognized, ignored, or misunderstood, now tries again to get some understanding, recognition and comfort. What happens quite often in either case is a completely unexpected refusal. The adult behaves as if he does not know anything about the previous excite-ment or rejection; in fact, he acts as if nothing had happened.
>
> (1969: 432)

He suggests that the older theory of trauma concentrated exclusively on the second phase, neglecting the existence of the other two. This new theory changes the basis of the theory of trauma from a quantitive consideration in a one-person psychology to the study of events in a two-person object relationship. He also suggests that

> this constellation may even throw some light on the dynamism of trauma in adult life, like explosions, aircraft or railway accidents etc.

It is very likely that in these situations the starting relationship between the individual and his environment. was confident and trusting, the accident struck him unprepared, destroying his trust.

However, this does not seem to explain the phenomena of shell-shock in battle and bomb-shock in air-raids, since it is difficult to conceive of the environment of the battlefield or air-raid as giving rise to an attitude of confidence and trust. Possibly both the quantitative and the object relational theories of trauma are necessary to explain all eventualities that give rise to traumas.

We can now proceed to a consideration of Balint's views on psychoanalytic training. His first venture into the topic of education was in 1938, in a paper called 'Strength of the Ego and its Education' (1939b), and in it he is concerned that ideas on psychoanalytic ego-psychology and psychoanalytic education (pedagogy) shall not be dominated by an emphasis on the role of the superego. He writes:

> Psychoanalytical ego-psychology has also largely been founded upon the study of obsessions and depressions. When more closely considered, it reveals itself as a psychology of dependencies, or, to put it differently, to a small extent as a psychology of the id, but in the main as a psychology of the super-ego. In it the ego itself becomes merely a battle-ground. As psycho-analytical ego-psychology and psychoanalytical pedagogy are almost of the same age, they have had a far-reaching influence on each other's development. From the beginning both have been dominated by an emphasis on the role of the super-ego.
>
> (*Primary Love and Psychoanalytic Technique*, p. 210)

This concern for the role of the superego in education is thought by Balint to be an important constituent in the various groupings that manifest themselves throughout the psychoanalytic world and is taken up in his next paper, 'On the Psycho-analytic Training System' (1948b).

Written in 1948, it constitutes a forceful criticism of psychoanalytic training. He first makes the point that up to this date, there is practically no literature on training, and that this is surprising since most training analysts are not averse to writing prolifically on other topics. He regards this lack of discussion of training as a sign of a severe inhibition and suggests that two possible reasons for this are, first, that criticism of training would imply that the older training analysts were not properly trained, and, second, that such discussion would also involve the efficiency or validity of analytic therapy in general. He also notes that the training analysts, as demonstrated by the procedures of the organization of training in psychoanalytic institutes, show a dogmatic attitude towards them 'unknown in any other sphere of psychoanalysis' (1948b: 5). He further believes that the general behaviour of analytic candidates is far too respectful to their training analysts. His conclusion is that the whole atmosphere is strongly reminiscent of the primitive initiation ceremonies in which

> the general aim . . . is to force the candidate to identify himself with his initiator, to introject the initiator and his ideals, and to build up from these identifications a strong super-ego which will influence him all his life. This is a surprising discovery indeed. What we consciously intend to achieve with our candidates, is that they should develop a strong critical ego, capable of bearing considerable strains, free from any necessary identification, and from any automatic transference or thinking patterns. Contrary to the conscious aim our own behaviour as well as the working of the training system have several features leading necessarily to a weakening of these ego functions and to the formation and strengthening of a special kind of super-ego.
>
> (1948b: 5)

Balint then examines the historical development of the training systems to see how this state of affairs arose and differentiated three periods of training.

> The first period of training was characterized by the lack of any visible organization – and there was no demand at a super-ego intropression, nor demand for a far-reaching identification. [Super-ego intropression is a term used by Ferenczi to denote a characteristic of some types of educative process where a rule or precept is forced into the super-ego. H.S.] This led to several secessions. In the second period psychoanalysis created an efficient system of training and a strong organization to enforce its standards. . . . By creating unnecessary tensions between the generations, this period led to recurring strifes and resulted in the complete breakdown of any central authority and in the establishing of local-national or group-standards, ideals, and controls. We start the third period having several claimants to loyalties in sharp competition with one another. This has led inevitably to a narcissistic over-valuation of small differences which in its turn blurred the real proportions by minimizing or completely hiding the essential agreements.
>
> (1948b: 8)

Nevertheless, Balint also adds that he believes that there are a very few hopeful signs that things are gradually changing and that general opinion among training analysts is veering towards the easing off of this superego training. However, six years later in his last paper on training, 'Analytic Training and Training Analysis' (1954a), he seems less optimistic about such changes. He now describes five periods in the history of training analysis.

> The first period was that of pure *instruction*, done mainly by the pupil himself, almost without any help from outside, simply by reading Freud's books. . . . This second period I shall call the 'period of *demonstration*' . . . a description of it given by Freud in 'Analysis Terminable and Interminable' (1937): 'For practical reasons this analysis can be only short and incomplete. . . . It has accomplished its purpose if it imparts to the learner a sincere conviction of the existence of the unconscious, enables him through the emergence of repressed material in his own mind to perceive in himself processes which otherwise he would have regarded as incredible, and gives him a first sample of the technique which has proved to be the only correct method in conducting analyses. . . . While the first two periods developed imperceptibly without any scientific discussion whatever, the third period, that of '*proper analysis*', was able to establish itself only after heated debates and the overcoming of considerable resistance. The protagonist . . . was Ferenczi, whose main argument, simplified to the bare bones, was that it was an untenable situation that the patients should be better analysed than their analysts . . . the fourth period started by the acceptance of another, still more exacting, demand, also by Ferenczi, according to which training analyses must achieve more than therapeutic analysis. . . . This 'fully completed analysis' is obviously more than is usually needed for therapeutic purposes, that is the reason why I propose to call it '*supertherapy*' . . . It is only in the last few years that some cautious people have rather timidly questioned the possibility of a supertherapy; they say that the aim of a training analysis is not its 'completeness' or 'proper termination' or 'supertherapy', but 're-search'. With that I have arrived at the last, the present, phase of our training system, which I propose to call the *period of research*.
>
> (1954a: 2)

Balint, in discussing supertherapy, recognizes that as there is no published scientific discussion of this topic, his own attempts to understand its dynamics will be subjectively biased. Furthermore, in this period the various schools and groupings emerged in the analytic societies, and since training is the most important way of propagating any particular set of ideas, it becomes involved in analytic power politics. He suggests that in the third period of 'proper analysis', the main interest was focused on the verbal expression of Oedipal complex material at a time when the child could express itself in words. In the next period of supertherapy, new techniques claimed to be able to reach pre–Oedipal states and to express non-verbal and pre-verbal experiences in words. He suggests that these new techniques consist 'of studying more and more finely and deeply the ever-changing phenomena of the day-to-day transference, and interpreting as many of its details as possible, especially in their aggressive-sadistic aspects' (1954a: 3). In discussing this, he makes two important points. The first is that

> too early and too consistent interpretation of slight signs of hatred may train the candidate to spare his analyst from and to protect him against the full brunt of fierce aggressiveness. Real hatred and hostility are only talked about, never felt and are eventually repressed by the taboo of idealization. If I may be allowed to use a colloquialism, the candidate is not able to nibble bits off his analyst, accepting some and rejecting others of his qualities, techniques and methods, because every such 'destructive' attempt could be interpreted and thereby prevented; the analyst must be 'swallowed whole', as a whole, ever repaired and idealized object.
>
> (1954a: 5)

The second point is that

> St Paul's conversion teaches us that introjecting a previously hated and persecuted object in idealized form may result in intolerance, sectarianism, and apostolic fury. Phenomena reminiscent of these states may be met with in many psychoanalytic societies. I suggest that the cause of all this is that the ambivalently loved and idealized, introjected image must be preserved at all costs as a good and whole internal object. In such a state any outside criticism – whether justified or unfounded – merely mobilizes all the forces of the pent-up hatred and aggressiveness against the critic, and for the protection of the training analyst, his technique, ideas, and methods.
>
> (1954a: 5)

He believes that these two unattractive consequences of the super-therapies prompted some training analysts to experiment with a technique that would avoid them, the aim being characterized by the name 'research'. He maintains that it is not quite clear who is the subject and who is the object of the research. He wonders whether, with the help of the analyst, it is the candidate who has to find out something about the deep layers of his mind, or whether it is the analyst who, with the help of his candidate, wants to find out something about the possibilities and limitations of his technique. He believes that the main thing is that the training analyst should divest himself of any semblance of omniscience inherent in a supertherapist, and that he should try not to give too many, too early and too well-digested interpretations, which possibly may prevent the candidate from making his own discoveries. The aim 'is to bring up babies who may be lean and perhaps less satisfied, whose interest is not restricted to "good food", but who are independent and even somewhat lacking in respect. In our sober moments we know that there is a price to be paid for all that, but at present we do not yet know what the price may be' (1954a: 6).

Forty years on from the writing of this paper, it is still not clear what this price might be since the supertherapies have not been replaced by research therapies. Perhaps the need for idealization is too strong a motive force for any institution or society.

6

Critiques and further developments

In this chapter I want to devote myself to the surveys and critiques of Balint's work that have been published, largely since his death in 1970. It is a regrettable fact that this highly innovative and creative work has to some extent not received the credit and acceptance that I believe it deserves. One of the main reasons for this, I believe, is that he has not given his readers sufficient clinical material to allow them to judge for themselves the correctness or usefulness of these theories. Most other major psycho-analytical writers have supported their theoretical views with the clinical evidence on which the theories are based, and this has critically helped the understanding of their theoretical positions. Balint has not done himself justice even though, to remind you, as early as 1932 he stated in his paper on 'Character Analysis and New Beginning' that 'without clinical ex-amples, any discussion of technique is useless'. He should have followed his valuable advice himself.

However, the relative absence of clinical illustration does not apply in the same degree to his applied work and there is no obvious reason for this discrepancy. It could be suggested that he became more interested in applied work to the detriment of the pure, but the evidence does not support this since (1) his writings in pure work continued up to his death, and (2) his writings on pure work lacked much clinical illustration from the beginning of his career as a psychoanalyst. It remains a mystery.

One unfortunate result of this deficiency of illustration in his pure work is that it tends to make his work less vital and interesting to read, and this is regrettable since in clinical discussions, both as a supervisor and seminar leader, he could be vibrant and dynamic in his understanding and concept-ualizing of clinical material. In his technique, he was a classical analyst, mainly concerned with understanding conflicts arising from the defensive ego structures against the id-driven derivatives. As a supervisor, he questioned all assumptions made in the course of my understanding and interpreting clinical material, and his suggestion to me concerning interpretation was that I should have two or three possible interpretations in my mind, so that if the first seemed to be incorrect, I could always try the others. It is not difficult to see that although this may have been relatively easy for the experienced supervisor, it was a more daunting task for the student being supervised. Nevertheless, he was very tolerant of my inability to match his performance. He, interestingly, was one of the few supervisors who stopped his students from using any case-notes of sessions during the supervision, since he preferred the student to give his own account of sessions in a more spontaneous fashion. He used this same technique with the general practitioners in his Balint groups. If one uses the analogy of wood and trees, using notes makes one see the trees more clearly than the wood, whereas spontaneous reporting produces the converse effect. Both methods have their advantages and disadvantages, and during my super-visions with him, he suggested that my second supervisor should be a Kleinian, as this would teach me about the details of the trees. I found this suggestion most helpful for my subsequent development as an analyst.

Another possible reason for the relative failure of his views to be accepted by other analysts may well have been their mistrust of therapeutic regression, especially the physical contact between analyst and patient. It seems too close to appearing to be seductive and this may well have caused a mistrust, not only of regression, but of all his theories. If this is correct, it is regrettable since regressive techniques need no physical contact, not even finger-holding.

Masud Khan (1969), in his paper on Balint's researches on the theory of psychoanalytic technique, has given a wide-ranging review of his work. The paper was written 'from a wish to bear witness and pay homage to the researches of a distinguished and creative analyst', and this he does in a positive frame of mind, expressing his agreement with most of Balint's work. Khan himself had written a paper entitled 'Dread of Surrender to Resourceless Dependence in the Analytic Situation' (1972), which itself dealt with problems of regression in analysis, showing his clinical interest in accepting and working with such states. He does, however, show some disagreement with Balint. The first disagreement concerns love, and Khan remarks that

> [o]f course, Dr Balint has his personal preferences, which are global and unshakeable, one of which is his very romantic notion of love as the beginning and end of all human desire and effort. The ultimate force which compels patients to keep at their analytic work is 'their wish, often unconscious, to be able to love free from anxiety, to lose their fear of complete surrender'.
>
> (1969: 238)

His use of the words 'very romantic notion of love' suggests that he does not entirely agree with the theory of primary object-love, nor with the theory of hate and sadism being secondary, reactive phenomena, but he does not state his own views on these topics.

His second disagreement with Balint concerns benign relationship.

> I think he tends to overlook the crucial role of the reparative drive in the patient towards the analyst and his setting. It is here that I have found Mrs Klein's work often most useful in recognizing the true meaning and direction of the patient's behaviour; that what the patient needed to be recognized was not only what his wishes were from what Dr Balint would call the primary object, but also what he wanted to offer to the primary object.
>
> (1969: 247)

From my own experience of working with regressed patients, I would agree with both of Khan's disagreements.

Stephen Morse (1972), in his paper 'Structure and Reconstruction: A Critical Comparison of Michael Balint and D.W. Winnicott', compares their respective contributions to structural theory; namely, Balint's theory of the 'basic fault shell', and Winnicott's theory of the true self–false self split. Morse's thesis is that, 'despite their use of different terminology, both theorists have constructed essentially similar conceptual frameworks to explain their essentially similar data found in their analyses of borderline and deeply regressed patients' (1972: 487). We shall remain with Balint. After giving an account of the theory of the basic fault, ocnophilia and philobatism, Morse suggests that the theory is 'insufficient' (as, incidentally, is his view of Winnicott's theory).

> Structurally, he [Balint] claims that the fault exists in the ego but it does not seem to be a structural split. It is simply some kind of deficiency state – a feeling that there has been a loss that must be made good. . . . Metaphors are used which suggest that the fault may be healed but that a scar is always left. My contention is that the basic fault concept makes little sense unless seen in the context of the shell and the core. . . . Balint seems to come to this position when he writes that the healing of the basic fault leads to the shedding of defensive armours. His concept of defensive character structure (ocno-philic and philobatic) used to defend against the anxieties caused by the failure of primary love and later by over-excitation and fear of punishment makes sense. It is not so much a question of the shell feeling or being false . . . rather, the shell is important because, having become rigid to deal with early anxieties, it prevents a full range of experiencing. Underneath the shell is the needy core, the basic fault. If its needs can be met, then the shell need no longer be so rigid.
>
> (1972: 497)

However,

> claiming that the goal of psychoanalysis is the shedding of defensive armours in order to allow the individual to reach himself clearly implies that there is some sort of split between the armour-self and the self that is to be reached . . . but this explanation is rejected. However, my contention is that unless a splitting metaphor is accepted, Balint's explanation becomes mere description and not theoretical metapsychology . . . probably the basic fault refers to the ego split into the bad as well as good aspects.
>
> (1972: 497)

He goes on, 'However, two structural considerations are implied. First, originally the ego is whole, unfaulted and undifferentiated. Second, differentiation of the areas of the basic fault and the Oedipus complex takes place partly by internalization of environmental reality, whereas no such internalization is needed for the area of creation to be differentiated' (1972: 497). These structural considerations of Morse are purely derived from Fairbairn's theories (1963), and it is to him that Morse has turned to remedy the suggested theoretical deficiencies of Balint and Winnicott. Balint does, however, give a structure to his concepts of ocnophilia and philobatism since he describes them in terms of a 'kind of introjection' (*Thrills and Regressions*, 1959a: 107). He has left no record of his opinion on Fairbairn's revised structural theory with its schizoid (splitting) mechanisms. However, what Balint does not simply accept is the Kleinian theory of the primacy of the paranoid-schizoid position with its innate splitting, projective and introjective mechanisms, since he regards the clinical observations on which this theory is based as containing secondary narcissistic features. This would make the theory one of a secondary state, since narcissism is always secondary, and he suggests that this state makes it secondary to his concept of primary love (1952a).

Jonathan Pedder (1976), in his paper 'Attachment and New Beginning: Some Links between the Work of Michael Balint and John Bowlby', gives an account of a female patient whose needs, when in a benign regression, seemed to be for a physical contact. In this instance, it manifested itself in the analyst's holding the patient's hand; he thought that this became an important new beginning for the patient. He links this non-verbal physical contact experience with attachment theory, summarized by Bowlby (1975) as 'conceived as a class of behaviour that is distinct from feeding behaviour and sexual behaviour and of at least as equal significance in human life' (p.296). However in 1985, Pedder, in an author's preface to his paper, writes, 'The technique used has not become a standard part of my therapeutic repertoire, and I have not handled a case in a similar way since. Perhaps I now rely more on the interpretative mode' (p.296). This issue of physical contact, as I have previously remarked, is an important one and I shall examine it more fully in this chapter.

John D. ('Jock') Sutherland (1980), in a paper entitled 'The British Object Relations Theorists: Balint, Winnicott, Fairbairn, Guntrip', examines the work of the four theorists and suggests that, in common, they all had an essential contribution to make. 'Instead of grafting the implications of relations onto a theory that started from a different standpoint, what the British group has done is to show that the development of the person has to be conceived as the progressive differentiation of a structure from a unitary matrix that itself interacts at a holistic personal level from the start' (1980: 858). Sutherland was well acquainted with Balint's work, particularly since he was the director of the Tavistock Clinic at the time Balint was working there and developing his fundamental group-style work with general practitioners, analysts researching brief psychotherapy, and so on. In discussing Balint's theoretical position on early object relationships, Sutherland adopts a similar critical stance to Morse; this is not unexpected since Sutherland was an analysand and champion of Fairbairn.

> Although Balint eschews any attempt at making an adequate theory, it is clear that the individual who escapes major trouble at this basic fault stage must have achieved a very important structural change; a fundamental epigenetic development.
>
> (1980: 832)

> He does not attempt to show in what way, for instance, the earlier developments might conclude with the Oedipal phenomena . . . we are not offered any views about the structural changes that must underlie the development of persistent patterns of behaviour such as ocnophilia and philobatism. Also, while hate is based in the struggle to overcome the oppressive dependence on the primary object and the giving up of primitive omnipotent wishes – he makes no reference to related structural concepts, e.g. of internal objects.
>
> (1980: 834)

My comment about Morse would also apply to Sutherland.

In their book *Object Relations in Psychoanalytic Theory*, Jay Greenberg and Stephen Mitchell (1983) devote a section to 'The Relational/Structure Models of Balint and Bowlby'. In giving a brief account of Balint, they state that 'Sensual, body-based gratifications are substitutive replacements for what is missing in terms of primary-love, derived from whatever partial contacts the parents are able to offer' (p.183). This is in referring to Balint's 'pre-genital organizations' paper of 1935. They then consider that 'Balint grants relational needs primary theoretical status', which they regard as taking him into a position roughly similar to Fairbairn's, yet, at the same time, continuing to maintain the drive/instinct theory.

> Although he has agreed that sensual strivings are derivative of relational needs, Balint alternately reinstitutes sensual pleasure-seeking as having primary motivational status in its own right. He chastises Fairbairn for abandoning libido theory, arguing that libido has two fundamental tendencies – that it is both pleasure-seeking and object-seeking. Thus despite his own reformulation of the nature and function of drive impulses, Balint continues to employ the term 'id' and the language of drive theory as if they had the same referents they have in Freud's work. Balint's critique of Fairbairn seems baffling in the light of his own redefinition of the pleasure-seeking aims of the libido as derivative of disturbances in object-relating.
>
> (1980: 183)

There is, however, a flaw in Greenberg and Mitchell's argument, since as far as I see it, Balint has not redefined 'the pleasure-seeking aims of the libido as derivatives of disturbances in object-relating'. Balint has consistently differentiated the development of pleasure-seeking aims of the libido from the development of object relations. Both are primary in their own right. However, some of the pleasure-seeking sensual body aims of the libido can become secondarily intertwined with those of the disturbed object relationships, as described by him in the pre-genital organizations paper, and this occurs because of the influence of cultural educational processes. In this way, only some of the sensual libido becomes secondary, not all of it; Balint may not have spelt out the processes in the amount of detail that we would have liked, but he has not been inconsistent or baffling in the way his critics suggest.

Greenberg and Mitchell next proceed to the idea that Balint held a position with regard to the dual nature of libido in order to try to resolve the dispute between Ferenczi and Freud over regressive techniques. They say that Balint distinguishes two types of regression, one of 'recognition' and fulfilment of primary relational needs, and the other of gratification of instinctual cravings; he also distinguishes psychopathology derived from disturbances in object relations (basic fault) from psychopathology derived from conflict (over instinctual wishes). They suggest that

> Balint's distinction does serve his larger political purpose, however. It allows him to preserve Freud's drive-structure theory and his wariness towards gratification (Freud was dealing with malignant regression, the pursuit of infantile instinctual gratification), while

justifying Ferenczi's focus on early object relations and his provision of gratification (Ferenczi was dealing with 'benign' regression in which relationship, not pleasure, is the goal).

(1980: 184)

This political agenda on Balint's part may or may not be the case, but since their argument is crucially based on Balint's 'baffling' use of the dual nature of the libido, which does not appear to be valid as I have already indicated, it is difficult to accept the validity of their own argument on this matter.

Lastly, there is the critique of Balint's work by Harold Stewart (1989) in his paper, 'Technique at the Basic Fault: Regression', which examines some of the technical problems encountered with patients regressed to the basic fault level. After a brief discussion of Balint's ideas, I state that:

Balint defined the problem as 'how to enable an uncooperative part of a patient, to cooperate, that is, to receive analytic help . . . a kind of reduction of his resentment, lifelessness, etc., which appear in his transference neurosis as obstinacy, awkwardness, stupidity, hyper-criticism, touchiness, greed, extreme dependence, and so on.' In my opinion this description is not strong enough as it does not encompass the sheer malice, destructiveness, and extreme envy that is also behind the lack of cooperation. Khan had previously made this point in his essay on Balint's researches.

(Stewart 1989: 223)

I would also say that in this mental state, the patient is not suffering a transference neurosis but a transference borderline psychosis.

In his clinical examples of patients at the basic fault, Balint gives only patients who are in a benign regression and none in a state of malignant regression. This absence of clinical material may leave readers of his work with the idea that in dealing with these states, his technique of 'unob-trusiveness' means that the analyst says almost nothing to his patient but sits passively as a 'primary substance' and endures everything. To counter-balance this view, two patients in a state of malignant regression are presented in this paper, and a further example suggested from a case of Masud Khan's (1972). Margaret Little's (1985) account of her regressive experiences during an analysis with Winnicott is also of interest in this respect, since it gives a good picture of Winnicott's technique, which, although similar in some respect to Balint's, allows for more gratifications and bodily contact between patient and analyst, often initiated by the analyst.

This brings us to the problem of physical contact in the analytic situation.

He [Balint] thought that in the context of an *arglos* atmosphere, this physical contact is not only acceptable but therapeutically helpful, and his experience that it did not seem to be addictive must have encouraged him in this belief. It is very important here to note that Balint was very much against allowing physical contact of any sort except in this context. My own experience of him very firmly forbidding me to hold or allow any hand contact with my first supervised training case during the second year of her analysis bears this out. In this respect he differed considerably from Winnicott. . . . Strangely enough, Balint seemed to sound a warning against touching in his previous book, *Thrills and Regressions*: 'I thought that the need to be near to the analyst, to touch or to cling to him, was one of the characteristic features of primary love. Now I realize that the need to cling is a reaction to a trauma, an expression of, and a defence against, the fear of being dropped or abandoned' (1959[a], pp.99–100). In the more recent literature, Casement (1982) gives a description of his patient's early traumatic experiences with her mother which emerged in the analysis when he refused to allow hand-holding; this confirms Balint's seeming warning. . . . I have noted, and so have some colleagues, that after allowing hand- or finger-holding, even though it is late in the analysis and in an *arglos* atmosphere, the patient will have a dream, frightening or otherwise, of being raped or sexually assaulted. The inference is that the unconscious experience of the patient had been very different from that of an innocent physical contact. My last point concerning the wish or need for physical contact is that I have only experienced such requests from female patients and never from a male, but perhaps this may be because my experience of treating male homosexuals is relatively limited.

My conclusion from these points is that although physical contact may be therapeutically useful, it may also conceal more than it discloses. Furthermore, it also makes me wonder about the nature of the *arglos* atmosphere. It could well be that on some occasions the atmosphere may seem to have this quality because the psychic realities of persecutory traumatic and sexual anxieties have been split-off and denied, leaving the opposite state of innocence and guilelessness in a hysterical-type defensive manoeuvre. As the analyst cannot differentiate the real *arglos* state from the fraudulent, it seems therapeutically more advantageous to forgo physical contact rather than risk colluding with the patient's denials.

(Stewart 1989: 226–7)

Interestingly enough, a letter written by Winnicott (1987) to Balint on 5 February 1960 seems to support this view of the *arglos* state:

I become more definitely in disagreement with you when you use the word harmonious in description of the relationship which you call primary love. As soon as the word harmonious is used I feel I do know that a highly complex and sophisticated defence organization is at work in the child who is no longer a newly born baby or a pre-natal infant.

FURTHER DEVELOPMENTS

The developments that have so far arisen from Balint's psychoanalytic work are in the realm of benign and malignant regression. Khan (1972), in his paper concerning a patient in a state of malignant regression, thought that this state was basically reactive to a dread of surrender to resourceless dependence in the analytic situation. He characterized the patients as coming from an over-protected environment in infancy and childhood, which did not allow for the aggressive behaviour that is essential for the crystallization of identity and separateness of selfhood in the child. He also noted the presence of severe destructive envy, which spoiled and negated any indication that the analyst's work had been helpful to the patient. My own experience supports his views on dread of surrender and of destructive envy, but I found that some of my patients came not from over-protected environments but under-protected ones, where the parents had been unpredictable, often violent, and often absent for prolonged periods.

Christopher Bollas (1987), in his book *The Shadow of the Object: Psycho-analysis of the Unthought Known*, discusses benign regression, or regression to dependence in Winnicott's terminology. He particularly discusses it in terms of the mental process of 'musing':

> Musing is part of the receptive ability, established as a valued part of the analysis by the analyst's capacity to receive the analysand during silent states. The capacity to receive, which enables the mental function of musing, may facilitate another mental process: evocation. Musing is formless, an aimless lingering amidst perceptual capacities, such as imagining, seeing, dreaming, touching and remembering. Evocation describes the passive state in which the more active elements from the unthought known arrive. [The unthought known is that which is known unconsciously but not yet thought.]
>
> The intersubjective process which facilitates this kind of regression depends upon the analyst's function as a transformational object, experienced by the patient in ways similar to the infant's experience of the mother: as an object associated with a process that does not distinguish between internal and external perceptions.
>
> The analyst's capacity to become part of this intersubjective process as a transformational object rather than as a separate object amounts

to an act of 'provision' within the countertransference; it enables the analysand to deconstruct ego functions in the interest of early states of self.

Recovery from regression emerges naturally as a result of the analysand's discovery of something pleasurable or inspiring, even if anxiety provoking, which he wishes to tell the analyst. There is then a need for the analyst's analytic function and a need for the analyst to engage in a discussion with the patient.

(Bollas 1987: 272–3)

Lastly, Harold Stewart (1989, 1992) gives his views on the subject of malignant regression. Balint believes that the analyst should try to prevent the development of a malignant regression by eschewing any technique suggestive of omniscience and omnipotence. I add

that interpretations in sexual terms concerning sexual phantasies and conflicts, if given early in the analysis or else when the patient is regressed to the basic fault level, can easily lead to mental states of overstimulation and overexcitement which may easily lead to severe acting-out in a malignant fashion. The third contribution the analyst can make to a malignant regression is to gratify the patient's wishes.

(Stewart 1989: 227)

Aspects of the technique of treating these cases are then discussed and these, briefly summarized, are:

1 the vital importance of maintaining the analytic setting and the analytic stance;
2 the necessity at crucial times for confronting the patient in the interest of maintaining the analytic setting;
3 the need to interpret the intensity and malignancy of the patient's destructive, envious attacks on the analyst's capabilities and capacities;
4 the need for the analyst not to confuse his own healthy aggressive firmness with his potential sadistic cruelty.

In 'Clinical Aspects of Malignant Regression', Stewart (1992) outlined a series of motivations that go to make up the state of a malignant regression. These are:

1 To obtain gratification of libidinal desire, particularly to fill chronic states of inner emptiness.
2 To spoil and destroy helpful good objects because of excessive envy.
3 To spoil and destroy helpful good objects so as to avoid the anxieties of dependence.
4 To spoil and destroy helpful good objects so as to avoid the anxieties of separation.

77

5 To test the analyst's ability to maintain the limits and boundaries of the analytic setting.

6 To test the analyst's ability to maintain the analytic stance under the most intensive provocation without retaliation.

7 If one accepts Winnicott's theory (1969) that destructive impulses create the reality of objectively perceived objects, this is an unexpected positive motive for a malignant regressive state.

(Stewart 1992: 40)

These motivations are illustrated by the clinical descriptions of the analysis of severe hysterical borderline patients that are given in Stewart's book and papers; together with this, there are further illustrations of states of benign regression and the occasional difficulties of differentiating between the two states.

From this overview of Balint's work and development, we get a picture of a man who could produce interesting, stimulating and provocative theories which sustained, and continue to sustain, the interest of many of his colleagues. He became an analyst in the early 1920s when Freud's theories were changing from their emphasis on the unconscious and its drive-derivatives to the study of the defences and the object in their relationship to his new structural theory. At this time, Ferenczi was particularly interested in the mode of functioning of the patient's object, the analyst, and the positive and negative ways in which that object could affect the functioning of the patient. This interactive object relationship became the centre of Balint's interests, and his theorizing attempted to accommodate the drive/defence theories of the one-person relationship with these interactive processes of the two-person relationship. Object relations theory, which is now taken for granted, had to be fought for, and Balint and his contemporaries, Klein, Winnicott, Bion and Fairbairn, were in the forefront of that struggle. Their work has continued among their successors and has inspired a great deal of new thinking. Balint's theories are very relevant today, particularly in the field of early interactive and intersubjective phenomena, and possibly, his theories in the analytically obscure area of bodily-sensual phenomena will yet lead to further developments. Balint was always open to new thinking in his colleagues, and the study of his work could act as a potent mental stimulus to anyone who values open-mindedness of thought.

It must, however, be said that, in its own terms, his theory of development is not completely satisfactory. He had introduced the concept of two lines of development, one of instinctual object-relations and the other of instinctual aims towards objects, yet his focus was almost entirely on the object relations line. This resulted in the relative neglect of the development of instinctual aims, but more crucially, it resulted in the neglect of the investigation of the relationships and connections between them. This has resulted in a lack of integration in this area, and it remains in need of further development.

This concludes Part One on pure psychoanalysis, which has presented Balint, the theoretical and technical innovator. Part Two is mainly concerned with his pioneering work with general practitioners, and Bob Gosling, Balint's colleague at the Tavistock Clinic, presents us, among other things, with a vivid picture of Balint's functioning and personality in the immediacy of his clinical and teaching groups.

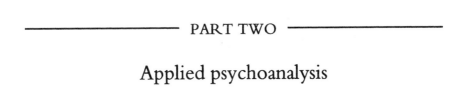

PART TWO

Applied psychoanalysis

7

Applied psychoanalysis

Balint, from his early years as a psychoanalyst in Budapest, had always been a keen exponent of the value of the application of psychoanalytic principles and insights to other fields of medical and social practice. Freud, in his paper 'Lines of Advance in Psychoanalytic Therapy' (1919), had been the first advocate of this use of psychoanalysis to help patients who, for many reasons, were unable to avail themselves of full analysis: 'the large-scale application of our therapy will compel us to alloy the pure gold of analysis freely with the copper of direct suggestion; and hypnotic influence, too, might find a place in it again, as it has in the treatment of war neuroses' (p. 168).

Ferenczi, too, had been interested in the psychological aspects of medical practice. André Haynal (1988) in his book *The Technique at Issue*, which discusses controversies in psychoanalysis from Freud and Ferenczi to Balint, states that 'he [Ferenczi] observes that "the personality of the physician often has a greater affect on the patient than the medicine prescribed". This observation is the point of departure for Michael Balint's ideas on medical education' (1988: 92). He further quotes Ferenczi as wondering 'How the future medical student will acquire this profound self-knowledge [of psychoanalytic sensitivity] is a difficult question to answer' (ibid. 92). He continues:

> By way of reply, Balint set up 'training and research groups for general practitioners', on the lines of the Hungarian psychoanalytic system. Before the development of the Berlin Institute's so-called 'tripartite' training system, which calls for personal analysis, courses on theory, and supervision, the Budapest school made no such clear-cut distinction between these three aspects of training. Hungarian candidates associated freely in their own analyses around the cases they were treating. Balint thought that it should be possible to create a training for general practitioners that would bring about a

limited though considerable change in the doctor's personality, allowing a better understanding of the doctor–patient relationship. Balint's premise was that any emotion felt by the physician in treating a patient should be considered a symptom of the illness.

(1988: 92–3)

This premise underlines much of Balint's applied work from the early 1950s, not only with general practitioners but also with marital therapists, family planning practitioners, and analysts working with brief psycho-therapy. It is the using of counter-transference responses, a powerful non-verbal communication from patient to therapist, as a vital source of information. It has been noted previously that Balint is one of the pioneers of the positive use of the counter-transference, and this is used in the various settings in which the therapy took place. These settings would be the surgery for the general practitioner, and the clinic, consulting room or hospital for the marital therapists, those specializing in psychosexual problems, and the brief psychotherapists. The therapist's basic discipline and training would determine the setting of the therapy.

Balint is connected with many of the innovations that were introduced into the practice and training of psychotherapy in this country. Apart from his researches in psychoanalysis, he started the general practitioner seminars at the Tavistock Clinic in 1950; started a brief psychotherapy workshop with analysts from the Cassel Hospital and the Tavistock Clinic in 1955; started seminars for the treatment of psychosexual disorders with the Family Planning Association; in 1949 started marital therapy seminars with the Family Discussion Bureau, later to become the Institute of Marital Studies at the Tavistock Centre; and in 1961, he started Balint seminars with undergraduate students at University College Hospital.

A most important outcome of these research seminars was a series of books written by the participants. Balint was the sole author of *The Doctor, His Patient and the Illness* (1957a), but in addition, he collaborated on a number of others with colleagues, particularly his wife, Enid. These are *Psychotherapeutic Techniques in Medicine* (1961) with Enid Balint; *A Study of Doctors* (1966a) with Enid Balint, Robert Gosling and Peter Hildebrand; *Treatment or Diagnosis: A Study of Repeat Prescriptions in General Practice* (1970a) with N. Hunt, D. Joyce, M. Mainker and J. Woodcock; and *Focal Therapy – an Example of Applied Psychoanalysis* (1972) with Enid Balint and P. Ornstein. He also inspired general practitioners to write on research topics of interest that had arisen in their groups. These include *Night Calls* (1961) by M. Clyne; *Virgin Wives* (1962) by L. Friedman; *Asthma, Attitude and Milieu* (1966) by A. Lask; *Sexual Discord in Marriage* (1968) by M. Courtenay; and *Six Minutes for the Patient* (1973) by E. Balint and J. Norell. Apart from Balint's own book on general practice, the books of David

Malan on brief psychotherapy, and particularly *A Study of Brief Psychotherapy* (1963), have become world-renowned classics in their respective fields.

The work with general practitioners will be discussed further on, but here we can consider his work on brief focal psychotherapy, sexual and marital therapy. Eric Rayner (1991), in his book *The Independent Mind in British Psychoanalysis*, having been an original member of the workshop devoted to brief therapy, gives an account of the work taking place in the group:

> In contrast to analysis, where the slow unfolding of emotional structures was allowed to proceed at the patient's speed, the aim of brief therapy was 'to go in fast, work at depth and come out quick', as it used to be put by members of the group. This needed the formulation of a clear, conscious plan of action from the outset. The therapist needed to be very well informed analytically to be able to detect unconscious structures. Optimally, he also needed to be monitored throughout by colleagues in order to maintain the confidence, clarity and consistency that the work demanded. The first essential requirement was psycho-diagnostic skill. Patients were always seen by a psychotherapist and a psychologist, both analytically trained. An assessment was made of the patient's predominant character structures and then, within this setting, of the nature of the unconscious conflicts which were centrally manifest and predominant in the current crisis.
>
> If a patient seemed to be of such a character that he was preoccupied by diffuse, amorphous, hence more-or-less objectless, long-term anxieties and was consequently prone to withdraw into his own self-deluding inner world, then brief therapy would not be indicated. The level of such problems could readily be diagnosed as 'at a one- or two-person level of functioning'. On the other hand, if a patient was worrying about conflicts that directly involved himself with other people and moreover was aware that he might be involved in playing a part in creating the problems, then brief psychotherapy would be more likely to be considered. . . . The assessment then proceeded by the reports of the two initial assessors being discussed by the workshop and a treatment plan being defined. This laid out the focus of conflict that seemed to be pressing and was thus readily available for brief work. The therapist was left free to carry out the treatment according to his own judgement but he had to record carefully every session and be able to be answerable to the group for his interpretations and actions. Close criticism was the norm in the discussions. This included the therapeutic work by Balint himself,

who could on occasion be subject to merciless criticism. Workshop decisions were evolved democratically.

(Rayner 1991)

Of course, outside of the setting of the workshop, hospital or clinic, the diagnostic assessment and treatment formulation would be made by therapists themselves, working on their own, but adequately trained in this type of therapy, which requires its own special skills.

In the book on focal therapy, we get a rare glimpse of Balint at work on a case, albeit as a focal therapist doing brief therapy rather than as a psychoanalyst doing analysis. Balint wanted to write this book on the technique of focal therapy in order to complement Malan's book (1963), which did not study technique but criteria of selection, outcome and follow-ups. The book is based on Balint's treatment of a paranoid, latent homosexual man who suffered from an abnormal preoccupation of his wife's feelings towards another man. Balint decided to offer him a brief focal intervention since he did not want an analysis, and there were twenty-seven sessions given over a period of about fifteen months. He kept systematic notes on each session, and this gives us a picture of his thinking and interpreting when functioning in this setting. An interpretative stance is maintained throughout the therapy, and any reassurance or advice is eschewed. The final outcome is very satisfactory and shows the potential benefits of this form of brief therapy. In the present climate of economic setbacks for full psychoanalysis, this work becomes of great importance in the analytically orientated treatments for mental and emotional ill-health.

In 1948, a seminar for social workers who were trying to develop techniques for assisting people in marital difficulties was started at the Tavistock Institute. It was called the Family Discussion Bureau and was headed by Enid Eichholz, the future Mrs Balint. In 1949, Michael Balint was asked to join the project, and together they developed the 'case discussion seminar'. They devised a method of parallel therapy of the two marital partners by two separate therapists, with the two therapists regularly meeting and being supervised by a third. The technique was developed and refined, and the Bureau became the Institute of Marital Studies.

In the early 1950s, Balint was asked to become a consultant to the Family Planning Association. This was an organization of doctors and nurses who were offering contraceptive advice and prescription, and they had discovered that emotional problems arose in the patients, particularly at the time of the physical examination. Balint responded by means of a workshop to discuss the problems and developed techniques for short focal work particularly at these critical moments, and in the course of time the Association became the Institute of Psychosexual Medicine. By any standards, this is a most impressive outcome from one man's research projects in applied psychoanalysis.

There are further developments in the field of applied psychoanalysis from the work of Enid Balint and the general practitioners of the Balint Society in the shape of three books, which continue the Balint tradition. The first is *Six Minutes for the Patient*, edited by Enid Balint and Jack Norell (1973), and it gives an account of the useful work that can be done in the six minutes, that is the time of the average general practitioner/patient consultation, by the understanding of the doctor–patient relationship. The second is *While I'm Here, Doctor*, edited by Andrew Elder and Oliver Samuel (1987), which is a further study of this relationship. Lastly there is *The Doctor, the Patient and the Group* by Enid Balint, Michael Courtenay, Andrew Elder, Sally Hull and Paul Julian (1993), which examines the developments in the groups from their beginnings in the 1950s and assesses the usefulness or otherwise of their features in the test of time. With Enid Balint's death in 1994, it will be of interest to see if this work continues to be developed in the absence of the Balints.

8

The general practitioner training scheme

ROBERT GOSLING

Michael Balint was the son of a general practitioner in Hungary, where he was brought up. He himself became a doctor and a chemist but then veered towards the study of psychoanalysis. In Hungary the psychoanalytic training was under the influence of Sandor Ferenczi and differed in some respects from what had become established in Vienna; in particular, the trainee's first clinical case was supervised by his own analyst and not by someone else outside the analytic situation, as was the practice elsewhere. This system naturally brought into the foreground the interaction between the two participants, the trainee analyst and his patient, including the counter-transference as well as the transference. By now, years later, this perspective, though not the method of training, has come nearer to being the norm in analytic practice than it was then.

As a consequence of the terrible events in Hitler's Germany he found himself in 1949, after some years in Manchester, on the staff of the Tavistock Clinic in London. At that time the Clinic had three principal preoccupations: a devotion to the furtherance of psychoanalysis and its social effectiveness; a long-standing tradition of providing post-graduate courses to a variety of mental health workers; and as a result of recent experiences in the armed forces an excitement about groups and their possible uses.

In the field of postgraduate training in general the Clinic staff had by then become increasingly disillusioned with the value of lectures alone. In the case of GPs, as a result of a traditional post-graduate course a doctor was inclined to go back to work considerably impressed by the sagacity of the lecturer but also uncomfortably oppressed by a sense of his own ineptitude; he had a head full of new ideas but no new skills. Balint decided that it was useless to go along this well-worn and largely useless path and that a scrutiny of the work of a GP in the light of psychoanalytic understanding was worth a try.

So it was in this context that Balint's latent wish to contribute to general practice began to take shape. His aim was to offer the GP an experience that might open up for him a new perspective wherein he could develop increased awareness and new skills. He also hoped to articulate some new concepts and theories that would help to make greater sense of a GP's working life.

The technique he introduced had its beginnings in a slightly different endeavour. Faced with our ignorance of the dynamics of the marriage relationship and the need to develop better methods for helping marriages in distress, Enid Eichholz, who later became Balint's wife, was convening a group of similarly concerned colleagues. In their efforts to get to grips with these issues she asked Balint to join them and to help in any way he could. This group was called the Family Discussion Bureau and was the forerunner of what is now the Tavistock Institute of Marital Studies, a greatly expanded and developed organization with a high reputation in its field. As an effective point of entry into their work Balint introduced the technique of studying the ins and outs of the relationship that developed between the marital partners and their professional workers in order to throw light on the complaints that had become established. As this had proved useful it encouraged both him and Enid Balint to try something similar with GPs. He came to call this kind of work by the inelegant name of Research-cum-Training.

The original group of GPs that started out with him in 1952 must have been a collection of the most unusual personalities. With nothing to go on but the declared aim of the seminar, they jumped in. Those who could jump in deep stayed the course, learned a lot, acquired new skills and produced the book *The Doctor, His Patient and the Illness*, though it was basically written by Michael Balint alone (1957a). Those who found the way the seminar developed not to their liking dropped out; though they thereby missed a great deal, they nevertheless had probably shown good judgement for themselves.

The findings of that first seminar as articulated in Balint's book were indeed discoveries. Inevitably, subsequent seminars were composed of doctors who had already read the book and who could therefore make a more informed, if not guarded, decision as to whether or not to join. They were not quite such abandoned explorers as those in the original attempt. Moreover, as more and more was discovered there was a greater tendency to pass on the information and thereby to short-circuit the experience of working one's own way through to a new realization. Nevertheless, with Balint around, the frontiers of understanding were forever being pushed further out. Since his time there has been a tendency to let up on the pressure for investigation and discovery and to slip into a more traditional teaching mode. A seminar engrossed in this kind of activity is emphatically not using 'the Balint Method'.

In this chapter his work in building the GP training scheme at the

Tavistock Clinic will be described from the point of view of group work. In the next, it will be examined from the point of view of psychoanalysis.

Quite early in the experiment a practical and effective way of working was evolved. A seminar consisted of between eight and twelve GPs, all of whom were actively involved in practice and had full responsibility for the treatment of their patients. They were serious about their work and were painfully aware of not being able to meet some of the needs of their patients through their ignorance and ineptitude. Doctors intending to go into general practice but not yet enmeshed in it were not welcome; nor were observers, unless they were psychiatrists who wished to learn the technique of leading such groups. The seminar was in those days led by a psychoanalyst who was usually, but not always, a psychiatrist as well; he might in addition have one or two associates with him to help in the task of leadership and in developing the technique of such leadership.

The seminar met regularly and weekly for one and a half or two hours each time. Although the contract was exploratory and open-ended there was a fair expectation that nothing substantially useful for the GPs would emerge for something like two years. This expectation was derived from therapeutic work and the time that it usually takes for real changes in attitudes and behaviour to take place as opposed to the learning of new tricks. As it turned out, for one reason or another, this expectation seemed to be borne out by experience. The way the whole training scheme developed up to 1965 is reviewed in *A Study of Doctors* by M. Balint, with E. Balint, R. Gosling and P. Hildebrand (1966a).

The subject for discussion was always a case-history that one of the GP members had on his mind, one that oppressed him, challenged him or amused him: it was one that in some way had got under his skin, whether painfully or otherwise.

The focus of interest on 'the case' was not primarily on its symptomatic or historical details, but on the doctor–patient relationship as it was being revealed to the seminar by the way the GP presented his account of 'the case'. The aim was to clarify what the doctor was doing to the patient in terms of emotional life and what the patient was doing to the doctor. The task of the seminar leader was to engage the interest of the GP members in doing this. The leader's opening remarks were always, 'Who's got a case?' At first the doctors, in line with their orthodox medical training, considered 'the case' to be a patient they had seen in their practice; gradually, as the work proceeded it became evident to them that in this seminar 'the case' was an account of a doctor-and-his-patient in interaction.

The work of exploration grew out of the other group members' responses to the case presentation; it was their observations, reactions and realizations in the here-and-now of the seminar that pushed the exploration on. And it was the leader's task to facilitate this in any way he thought appropriate. Although early in the life of a seminar there was always a compulsion to keep the proceedings in line with the decorum and insincerity usual in such professional meetings, what gradually developed was much more of a rough and tumble. At times one might become alarmed at the amount of turmoil Balint's leadership encouraged, but he was once heard to say, 'Don't worry. To be a GP you have to be as tough as old boots!' In fact his evident expectation that 'you were man enough to take it on the chin' showed the great respect he had for his GP colleagues and roused them to further efforts. For the faint-hearted it also revealed the implied condescension in his protectiveness towards them. Balint's sincerity in considering the GPs themselves the best judges of the effectiveness of their work was demonstrated by his emphasis on the value of making mistakes in the learning process: although evident mistakes were to be deplored, their contribution to new learning was just as great as the occasions when the GP appeared to have got things right. It was a genuine, shared exploration of unknown territory – unknown in so far as this approach had not been tried before, in addition to the fact that the personality of each working GP was different and unknown. He made it quite clear that the leader was in no position to teach the GPs how to conduct their practices.

The relevant language that developed out of this was one concerned with how people treat one another – the different and changing relationships they sustain, in the past and in the present and in all likelihood in the future – with all its emotional consequences. The language was therefore more akin to object relations theory than to classical Freudian psychology. Indeed, if technical terms for intrapsychic function started to be bandied around the suspicion grew that some emotional difficulty was being avoided.

By the time that several such seminars had been running for a year or two a very general pattern in their development became apparent. When a seminar started there was a natural expectation that it would resemble the kind of undergraduate or postgraduate occasion the GPs were accustomed to. Indeed, for a while there was a considerable effort made by the GPs to reconstruct such a familiar occasion despite the rather uncooperative behaviour of the leader. An attempt was made to support the idea that the leader was an expert in what they had come to learn about, that he would hand over some of his expertise to them and that they themselves were safe from any unpredictable or painful experiences except those that might arise from the usual rivalry for the teacher's approval. In struggling to recreate this familiar configuration the GPs fell into their individual characteristic roles: the bright boy, the buffoon, the ingénu, the tough guy and so on, all well rehearsed from years of orthodox medical training.

Before long, however, the members had got so little support from the leader in this enterprise that they became frustrated and thoroughly disillusioned about him. This process was usually highlighted when a GP brought the case of a long-standing psychiatrically disturbed patient and the supposed expert turned out to be no more potent than anyone else. Provided the GPs did not give up in disgust at this point and could tolerate this degree of frustration they gradually came to value the observations that their fellow GPs could make: at least these colleagues were familiar with their working conditions and shared their desire for greater understanding. What became apparent was that there were many different ways of conducting general practice according to the strengths and limitations of the personalities of the various GPs. They began to learn from one another and to try out ways that others had shown them. At some point one was likely to hear a GP declare, 'Much to my surprise, with this patient I found myself doing a Dr Smith . . . or Brown, etc.'.

Inevitably, in this atmosphere a GP would at some time have the experience of having himself made the most useful observation and comment in the whole discussion. This would bring home to him that if anyone was a specialist in general practice it was the GP himself; furthermore, that there was no right way of conducting general practice, only the best way available for the particular pair concerned, the GP and his patient. As a result of this shift, the morale of the group improved a great deal and members were ready to push on further into areas that were worrying or obscure to them.

Every effort was made by the leader to keep the culture of the seminar clearly in the tradition of professional education and to prevent it slipping into the mode of personal therapy. To this end the seminars were always referred to as one of the numerous other training activities of the Tavistock Clinic and not part of its psychotherapeutic service. In addition, revelation in the seminar of a GP's emotional reaction to a patient, his countertransference, was acknowledged and worked with in the service of his professional endeavours but not as an important element in his personal life. Comments on a GP's counter-transference to his patient or his transferences within the group to other members or to the leader that were relevant to the task in hand were legitimated by the leader's behaviour and thereby given public status in the culture of the group. The extent to which these same emotional tendencies affected the GP's personal life was no business of the seminar. The leader had at times to be quite forceful in diverting the group away from its fascination with these personal issues and towards matters that lay within the concern of the doctors at their work. If a GP's wish to explore the ramifications of these reactions into his private world persisted, then he was told to seek a therapeutic relationship elsewhere. Invariably, the interactions in the group produced changes in the doctor's awareness of and reactions to people beyond the confines of his surgery, and to the extent that he received some therapeutic benefit he received a bonus. But the success or otherwise of this method of training was to be judged entirely by whether or not the GP's skill was enhanced in his daily work.

As a pointer to the kind of discussion that developed in the course of the original seminar one cannot do better than to list some of the catch-phrases that became current and were later elaborated in Balint's book: 'the drug "doctor"', 'the collusion of anonymity between GP and specialist', 'the apostolic function of the GP', 'having the courage of one's own stupidity', 'a limited though considerable change in the GP's personality', and so on.

Given the stated aim of the seminars as research-cum-training for general practitioners and given their setting in the Tavistock Clinic of its day, the way the method developed was principally a function of Michael Balint's preoccupations and his style of leadership. His approach to this new task was more that of an adventurer or sportsman than a classroom teacher; the atmosphere he created was nearer to that of a mountaineer's bivouac or a tennis court than to that of a lecture theatre; he expected people to exert themselves and to go home feeling stretched and stimulated. He was an attractive man: highly intelligent, vigorous, enthusiastic, challenging and provocative. Counter-dependency was his preferred stance: he could not abide colleagues toeing the line or mouthing what they had been taught. In this respect he much preferred the rough and tumble of his GP seminars to the more sycophantic atmosphere of some parts of the psychoanalytic world. Lecturing was not to his taste; instead he enjoyed being a stimulant to growth, even an irritant.

This quality was widely recognized, and resulted in his being made visiting professor to a number of educational institutions overseas where, during quite a brief stay, he would set a process of discovery and self-review going that left participants eager for his return. His challenging attitude invited rivalry, and when it was not too maddening to bear resulted in a good deal of independent thought. The number of topics researched and the number of resulting papers and books published by members of the seminars is impressive.

The stance he took up against slavish acceptance of other people's ideas had another side to it. Despite his challenging style he certainly needed to have round him a team of people who supported not only his aims but also his way of pursuing them, not necessarily people who agreed with what he said but people who would at least stand up to him on the basis of their own experience and not on the basis of some received 'truth'. This trait sometimes went further than he consciously intended and resulted in his having some sworn enemies as well as devoted followers. In fact he had very little time for those who did not want to go along with him.

By now it is well known that for groups to lead to changes in attitudes among the participants as opposed to changes in their conceptual furniture, it is the behaviour of the leader, his attitude to the task and the way he treats the participants, that count for more than the ideas he promulgates. It is therefore relevant to consider what the model was that Balint offered his GP colleagues by his behaviour.

Above all, he offered a model of someone who listened. He listened to everything that went on – to the preamble, to the story as it unfolded without interruption, to the asides, to the unconsidered remarks and to the jokes. But he did more than listen to the words that were said; he also took in everything that went on in the here-and-now of the session – the silences, the glances, the atmosphere – and then tried to make some sense of it all. He gave an example of someone seriously attending to what was going on in the seminar at the time the so-called history of the case was being presented and was having its impact on the other members. The verbal account of 'the case' was not enough; it had to be understood in the light of the emotional resonances that it set up. Peripheral thoughts and group associations of every kind were to be taken as seriously as any other more formal information that was offered. The attention to detail was great, but was not confined to conventional clinical matters. It was more like understanding a friend's predicament over and above the actual words he was using than taking the clinical history that medical students are taught to extract from bewildered patients.

The second important aspect of the model he offered was his firm adherence to the boundaries of his task. As mentioned above he was eager to know of the doctors' emotional responses to the cases discussed, but only in so far as they illuminated the clinical picture; efforts to carry them further into the private worlds of the doctors were resisted. In this way he gave a model of being open to as full an understanding as possible without being felt to be intrusive or meddling. In addition, by the language he used he kept a firm boundary between the world of general practice and that of psychiatry; the vocabulary he legitimated was that of the GPs describing their experiences with their patients, and he resisted so far as he could the intrusion of psychological terms from his own specialist background.

A third aspect of the model he offered proved to be more problematical: he was an irrepressible psychotherapist himself and would give clear signs of encouragement to those GPs who wanted to embark on 'long inter-views' of the kind used by professional psychotherapists, involving verbal confrontation and interpretation. To some extent this led to a premature invasion of the domain of general practice by a model appropriate to another setting. Gradually, however, he learned that here was another boundary that needed to be more closely monitored than his natural enthusiasm for psychotherapy had indicated.

By 1961 a number of psychoanalytically trained colleagues had joined Balint in this work and had taken on the leadership of such seminars both within and beyond the Tavistock Clinic. He therefore initiated a programme of staff seminars where the task of leading GP seminars could be explored among colleagues having this concern in common. It became an important reference group for those who attended – to say nothing of the pleasure of meeting once a month in the Balints' sitting room with coffee and cake to boot. Michael Balint led this staff seminar again in his own characteristic way. The subject matter of the meeting was provided by a pre-circulated verbatim record of a session of one of the participants' GP seminars. Other staff members were then encouraged to respond to it in as open and forthright a way as possible. In the early meetings there was of course a good deal of caution and circumspection in what was said. But by degrees, as participants became more secure with one another, just as in the GP seminars themselves, the atmosphere became more open and the comments made more far-reaching. Participation in this staff seminar was hard work, often stressful and immensely stimulating to thought in general and to the re-evaluation of one's own style and prejudices in particular. It was one of the most creative activities the author has ever engaged in.

Effective his style of leadership certainly was, but he was never heard to speak of how he thought he did it or how the consequent dynamic in the group assisted the learning of new attitudes and new skills. He was not much interested in the topic of group dynamics as such; he was simply an adept practitioner!

By this time, too, interest had grown in other parts of the world in Balint's way of working with GPs, and so several small international conferences were organized where others actively engaged in this sort of work could meet to discuss their common concerns. The form these conferences took was also greatly influenced by Balint's way of engaging with a group, and so there was a good deal of friction and a fair amount of learning.

What, then, was the result of this increasing institutionalization of his exploratory efforts? To some extent it led to an attenuation of the research component of his original intention. As more of the psychological features of general practice became articulated, in the publication of his book *The Doctor, His Patient and the Illness* in particular, the more the programme became suffused with a sense of things having been discovered that could now be taught. Of course, unforeseen features of general practice were still being discovered and every new GP and every new seminar leader still had the whole world, as it were, to discover for themselves; but an element of teaching certainly became more prominent among the efforts of Balint's associates even if it did not in his own work.

The staff seminar did, however, promote a good deal of useful understanding in relation to the use of groups in the furtherance of professional development in general and led to more refined work in seminars with a whole range of mental health workers. It also threw into relief the advantages and disadvantages of the seminar leader being of the same or different professional discipline as the seminar members. Although when the leader comes from the same stable as the members they will be familiar with the field under discussion, they will also to some extent be a captive of the assumptions and values of that particular discipline and so poorly placed to promote new thinking. Furthermore, their seniority and expertise may cast a shadow over the fumblings of the members and make it all the harder for them to make their own discoveries, often discoveries of things they have dimly known all along but had never allowed themselves to recognize and make use of. The growth of one's own awareness and confidence to use it depends upon renouncing to some extent the belief that one can gain it by looking to someone else; the importance of this other person has in some way to be diminished in one's mind.

When, say, an experienced old psychiatrist is leading a seminar of young psychiatrists, it would be a loss of a sense of reality if they did not think that were he in their shoes he might tackle the problem under discussion better than they could, and this might put their sense of their own efforts rather in the shade – whereas in a seminar of social workers a member's belief that this psychiatrist could do better than that member would have to be gradually exposed as a comfortable delusion, as an unresolved element of the Oedipus complex! A training by apprenticeship has many advantages but it is bound to encourage to some extent a spurious orthodoxy. Freedom to think for oneself always requires a struggle, but the struggle may be easier if the leader is more interested in the process of struggling than in whether what is arrived at is something that they approve of or not. This matter has been elaborated further elsewhere (Gosling 1978).

From the beginning it was evident that his way of working did not suit everyone, whether GP or psychiatrist; some found it too abrasive, disorderly and revealing. Likewise, the seminar leaders found there were some GPs who were so well defended against experiencing unexpected emotions that they acted as too much of a brake on the seminar for it to be profitable to engage with them any longer. Some left of their own accord out of frustration; others stayed on fighting doggedly and had to be ejected. It was never supposed that this way of working and the various personalities involved in it would meet the needs of all GPs across the board. A certain amount of 'fit' had to be there for much to come of the enterprise. In this respect a possibly useful model was provided for GPs in connection with their own expectation of themselves in relation to the wide range of patients they are expected to care for.

But for those who stayed, what did they gain from it? Essentially they developed two aspects of their personalities that had got neglected or even suppressed by their previous training: they became more aware of themselves and of the people they dealt with, and they gained a greater sense of authority for the work they were doing. The seminars helped them to recover from some of the side-effects of their medical education: to regain the ordinary sensitivity to people's emotional experiences that they had had before they became 'medicalized', and to acknowledge the value of the observations they could make as a result.

This awakened sensitivity usually began to stir when they discovered to their surprise that their own most 'unprofessional' and unwelcome feelings about a patient in fact threw some light on the patient's personality and recurrent stresses. They then began to feel more at home with their own emotional responses to patients and to value them as a possibly useful component of their diagnostic skill. In comparing their own reaction with that of other GPs in the seminar they also began to get a clearer view of their own peculiarities and propensities, and this led them to a greater appreciation of the variety of personalities to be found amongst both the GPs and their patients. As they felt more accepting of themselves they found they were more open to their patients and so began to understand them better; they found they could listen more easily and so became more interested in the problems that confronted them.

In parallel with this development they also found that they had a much wider range of possible responses to their patients than formerly. Some of these were released from their own resources and others were found through contact with their fellow GPs. In the course of this development there were, of course, episodes of incautious acting-out on the part of the doctors; but by degrees they learned to use more judgement in the pursuit of their professional work. This process of acquiring professional discretion was reinforced by the firmness with which the seminar was held to its primary task of professional development as distinct from personal therapy.

The second major gain from the seminars underpinned all the other changes, including the ones mentioned above, and involved a hard struggle with the Oedipus complex. Many of the doctors coming forward for these seminars were deeply convinced that 'real' medicine was the kind that they had learned during their hospital training and that they had seen exemplified by their specialist teachers. Their minds had become inhabited by these impressive figures as compelling role models for themselves. But in the course of their work in general practice they found that they could behave in that way only rarely and that they were poorly trained for most of the work that confronted them. They consequently felt like second-rate doctors and visualized 'good medicine' being practised elsewhere. In fact, it turned out that the most frequent time for a GP to apply to join a seminar was seven years after he had finished his hospital training. It seemed that by that time he was becoming disillusioned with his own work and his prospects. Several said that they were considering emigrating to 'new pastures' at the time but thought they would give the seminars a try!

In the seminar this shift of emphasis began when the effort to promote the leader into being a know-all and a dispenser of wisdom began to founder. In their frustration the GPs began to pick up the pieces and to turn to one another for help. In this atmosphere it came home to them that the only people in the room who knew how to practise medicine in the setting of families were they themselves; their knowledge might indeed be inadequate, but it was only they themselves who could extend it usefully. The leader might or might not be able to contribute an insightful remark, but whether to use it and if so how to use it were entirely matters for their own judgement. The leader made every effort not to get drawn into a collusion with the GPs that would attenuate their sense of their own full professional responsibility for the way they treated their patients. With varying degrees of success the GPs gradually came to know that they themselves were specialists in family medicine and that their teachers and hospital colleagues could be of use to them at their discretion but were irrelevant as judges of their performance. This shift of power from the superego to the ego invariably led to a considerable release of energy, enthusiasm and curiosity in their work. They usually forgot their plans to emigrate!

The value of this training scheme can only be judged by its results in terms of an enhancement of a GP's professional skills. The most general result of the seminars was that the GPs began to enjoy their work more and to feel they had more to contribute to it. Some seemed to change their overt behaviour very little – at least so far as they reported it. But it is hard to believe that their patients did not feel better cared for now that their doctors were enjoying their work with them and not just putting up with them while they longed to get away to the golf course. In addition, now that the GPs were less dominated by the values of hospital medicine and the primacy of 'cure', they could take more pride in themselves as they struggled over time, up hill and down dale, to 'care' for their patients and their families. And surely this would have been experienced as a great change by the majority of their patients.

Others, however, used their greater awareness of their patients' emotional lives to widen their range of responses which they could now use with greater discretion: to be permissive, decisive, encouraging, freely available, challenging, sharp and so on according to what seemed to be appropriate. They became less stereotyped in the way they behaved. A fair number also developed a capacity to talk with their patients in a way intended to throw light on the predicament the patient found themselves in, a form of psychotherapy adapted to the setting and the GP's personality.

There were many varieties of this development; most involved more confrontational moves than interpretations, though a few GPs became practised psychotherapists and even psychoanalysts after further training. The core of the methods used was to help patients to examine themselves rather than to expose themselves to being examined by the doctor.

Early in the programme it was Balint's hope to find a form of brief psychotherapy that was feasible for those GPs inclined to use it, and considerable time was spent in trying to work this out. What at that stage was being aimed at was something like the skills of a professional psycho-therapist. But despite Balint's enthusiasm for this, it proved to be inappropriate except for a very few; the majority adapted this model to a whole range of interventions of a reflective or confrontational kind that fitted in with the more intermittent contacts over a very long time that are typical of general practice.

The range of skills developed by the GPs is very considerable as can be seen from some of the many reports coming out of the seminars: for example, Hopkins (1960), Clyne (1961), Clyne *et al.* (1963), Lask (1967b), M. Balint *et al.* (1970a), E. Balint and J. Norell (1973), and Elder and Samuel (1987).

A notable result of this work has been the founding of the Balint Society, an association of all those interested in preserving this approach and in extending its uses. It is centred on the conduct of general practice in a changing world and is run by committed GPs themselves. Unfor-tunately, the present author is not in a position to give an up-to-date account of its achievements.

Concurrent with Balint's work at the Tavistock Clinic and later at University College Hospital in London and privately, many important changes were taking place in the field of general practice in Great Britain. The most important was the founding of the Royal College of General Practitioners which has given public recognition to the special skills needed for this kind of work in contradistinction to those needed in a hospital out-patient department. It has given sanction to the idea of family doctor-ing and has successfully pressed for increased numbers of ancillary staff working alongside the GP, so allowing a wider range of responses to be made to the patients' complaints.

Of great significance for the future is the increased time and emphasis given in medical schools to the problems and techniques of general practice and to the coherent post-graduate training in general practice that is now required before a young doctor can become a principal in a practice. It is said that increasingly the brighter students are now opting for general practice rather than for the glamour of hospital specialities.

It is certain that Balint's work played an important part in bringing about these changes. One only has to note the frequency with which important figures in the College and in GP training schemes are old members of his seminars to recognize his influence on the whole field.

Of course he was also a child of his time and was therefore influenced by and contributed to the concurrent changes in the intellectual climate. He had no option but to play a part in the paradigm shift that we appear to be experiencing from a more reductionist, mechanistic, Newtonian tradition towards a grappling with causal networks, systems theory, ecological and holistic concepts, and so forth. In psychoanalysis this is reflected in the displacement of drive theory by object relations theory. In this cultural climate Balint's work has made three contributions to general practice in particular: he has helped to bring to bear a perspective and some concepts that have thrown new light on a GP's work; he demonstrated that a degree of emotional involvement is required if these are to be used effectively; and he devised a method of training that permitted this to happen.

9

GP training and psychoanalysis

ROBERT GOSLING

What has this work with GPs to do with psychoanalysis? Certainly it is hard to believe that the approach would have been worked out except by someone experienced in psychoanalysis and deeply committed to its method and values. Doubtless, others can now get a firm grip on the technique and so can function as effective leaders of seminars. Indeed, the majority of such seminars in the United Kingdom are now led by experienced GPs who have taken part in this kind of work and not by psychoanalysts at all, though the extent to which they have moved away from the original 'Balint Method' is not known. But to make such a break with the long-standing tradition of postgraduate professional training, to eschew any ordinary kind of 'teaching', and to have carried the project through despite initial opposition from the members of the group and scepticism from psychoanalytic colleagues must have required a faith in the approach that could only have been acquired from a personal experience in another setting. Whether or not, however, this task could have been carried through by someone with a different background, we can nevertheless profitably scrutinize Balint's work from the point of view of psychoanalysis.

The salient characteristic of the Balint Method is that it is an exploration – an exploration of how things are between a certain GP and a certain patient at a certain time, and of the factors that have played a part in bringing this state of affairs about. This approach is epitomized in the title he gave to the project from its beginnings, namely, Research-cum-Training. In so far as any teaching crept in it did so adventitiously and almost despite his best efforts. When the demand for psychological theory became clamorous he arranged some didactic sessions at another time.

It was, however, a training as well as research and so presumably the GPs learned some skill that they did not have before. What they learned was an approach, a new way of looking at what had been in front of them all the time, one that involved attention to formerly ignored features of the situation including their own reactions to it.

What this new way of reflecting on their work would give any given GP would be peculiar to his own personality and stage of development: each GP had to make his own discoveries. There was, of course, a good deal of sharing of discoveries among members of the group, but there was very little pressure on anyone to accept what someone else had found unless it seemed to fit in with where one was at the time; it had to fit like a piece in a jigsaw puzzle.

In his approach to what went on in the group Balint communicated a deep conviction that the *unconscious mind* is always at work in all of us, not just in our patients, and that because of this there is always more to learn, more to surprise us, and therefore more channels for our development. This approach went hand in hand with a sincere respect for the GPs and the near-impossible job they have chosen to do with the limited resources available to them in terms of their external conditions, their training and the limitations of their own personalities. But his attitude also communicated a conviction that there were barriers that stood in their way that could be overcome through greater awareness of what they were dealing with. Readers must judge for themselves how closely this corresponds to the atmosphere analysts hope to establish in their consulting rooms.

The attention he gave to all the unconsidered remarks in the group, the jokes and the asides, the non-verbal communications made through posture, facial expression, silences, fidgetings and so on clearly stemmed from the experience he had had in the analytic situation with its reliance on *free association*. In a group situation, however, the exercise of *free-floating attention* is only possible from time to time. So much is going on and from so many directions that the leader usually feels caught in the middle of a bewildering cross-fire. Nevertheless, there are usually some moments of peace to be savoured when to drop out of activity into abstraction and reverie is possible. On such occasions, when a new and useful perspective on the matters in hand was found in this way, the GPs got some encouragement for taking a less blinkered approach to their own work. This more open receptivity when used in their own practice allowed the GP to entertain possibilities that had been excluded by their earlier medical orientation, such as to hear in a patient's 'history' an element of a cautionary tale about what may be expected to develop in the GP's own relationship with the patient, or to detect that the problem of a child's health may be the only way a mother can find a way to get in touch with her own desperation, or to realize that the patient who hangs back to be seen last at an evening's surgery is asking for more time to be spent with him even though that patient is initially unaware of this longing, for example.

Balint's relentless encouragement of the group members to explore further the predicaments they found themselves in without recourse to premature closure for the sake of their peace of mind, and his refusal to take over when things got difficult or to offer spurious reassurances, stimulated the GPs themselves to encourage their patients at times in the same direction – namely, to think more deeply about their own predicaments. Balint expounded this reorientation of the doctor's more usual relationship with patients in a paper entitled 'Examination by the Patient' (1960b) – that is, in contrast to the usual situation in which patients expose themselves to be examined by the doctor. This shift clearly stemmed from his recognition of the centrality of the *therapeutic alliance* in analytic work.

When a GP came forward to join this Research-cum-Training it was immediately evident to him that this was no post-graduate course of the usual kind. The commitment of time alone that he was threatened with was quite exceptional, and indicated that something quite different was envisaged from the usual passive absorbing of information. GPs found that it was they who were going to do the work and that the work required their emotional participation. The message came through with increasing force that developing interpersonal awareness and skills takes time and involves ups and downs and a whole range of responses, including backtracking and repetitions. The acceptance of this, indeed the expectation of it, and the active interest in it came from the experience in analysis of *working-through*, which is never boring unless a mode of teaching begins to take over. On the one hand this resulted in the 'limited though considerable change in the doctor's personality', and on the other an expectation that the GP's patients might also be able to make greater use of their contact with their doctor over a long period of time, a situation which is typical of general practice.

Although all the members had had similar medical trainings and so had been well schooled to defend themselves against emotional disturbances associated with their work and so, as a consequence, frequently tried to talk about their patients as if they were mechanical objects, Balint's focus was always where emotions were stirred in the group, either overtly or by their conspicuous avoidance. It was at this point, he believed, that further exploration might shift the perspective from the established one that had already proved of limited usefulness. The doctor presenting the case would be required to put his notes aside and to tell the story as it came to him; if the other group members persisted in searching for more details or engaged one another in an apparently learned discussion, he would try to refer the group back to the point where it had taken flight by asking them to reflect on what they had heard so far. It was at the point where emotions were active in the *here-and-now* that he believed useful work could be done. It was not that the patient's history, or personal myth as some might call it, was considered irrelevant; it was that it was not to be used as a retreat from the point of anxiety in the present.

The use the GPs made of this feature was very varied. In general it released them from the obligation to be clever and to say all-inclusive and recondite things; it freed them to believe that their own heartfelt but reasoned responses to the situation might guide them in their efforts to help their patients. It enabled them to tolerate the fact that any diagnosis they could make was usually little more than a working hypothesis, but to believe that they could yet be of considerable help to their patients – often of far more help than that provided by the impressive technical language of a specialist's report. It breathed life into what otherwise had become a bafflingly dead-end situation.

Balint's leadership was always challenging: it challenged some of the assumptions underlying medical practice and he challenged all about him to think afresh, maddening as it often was. In particular, when working in a GP group he took it for granted that the members would have to put up with a fair amount of frustration and exasperation if they were to make significant discoveries. The work he did was always in the setting of some *libidinal frustration*, whether this was for a dependent relationship with the leader or a collusive relationship with one or more peers. The frustration prevented the group from sinking into a self-satisfied complacency and provoked enough fury to stimulate the members' curiosity and deter-mination – in most cases! Where in analysis libidinal frustration is used to fire the patient's resolve to confront the infantile substrate of their personality that is thereby aroused, in the GP group it was used to confront the habitual medical defences that the doctors had so painstakingly acquired and which in many cases suited them so well. He would resist their regressive longings for authoritative pronouncements from the leader very firmly, and steadfastly maintained the boundary of his role despite all kinds of seductive manoeuvres.

The use of *interpretations* in the group as understood in psychoanalytic circles was always a vexed question. There was general agreement among the staff, however, that interpretations were only relevant in so far as they might further the task of exploring the doctor–patient relationship in question. Most of the leader's interventions, therefore, would be aimed at helping the GPs to put their various observations together in some way to make sense of what was going on between the doctor and his or her patient. This understanding would be tilted in the direction of clarifying the patient's more obvious predilections and conflicts in so far as they were playing an important part in the dynamic of the 'illness'. So the leader's interventions might be said to be leading the group towards formulating an interpretation, without, if possible, supplying one himself. But this was not an interpretation in the here-and-now, except in so far as the GP concerned had inevitably presented something of himself to the group while des-cribing his case.

The main point for discussion in the staff seminar was on when and how interpretation in the here-and-now might be used. *Confrontation* was certainly used when it seemed likely that what was going on in the group would throw some light on the case – for example, that the women doctors present seemed to have been silenced, which might suggest that the group had not noticed how much the patient under discussion had succeeded in excluding women from contact with their doctor. But the question as to how far this should be carried forward into an interpretation remained a vexed one; for instance, that the men in the group seem to be quite happy with this and the women seem to have got used to putting up with it. At this point some leaders would shift the focus back to the there-and-then of the doctor–patient relationship, and suggest, for example, that the patient was seeking a close and exclusive relationship with their doctor, or that they were afraid of or angry with women. It was generally hoped that the capacity to generate such thoughts and to hold them in the mind as possibilities would develop, but there was no agreement on how much should be fed in by the leader or should be left to arise from the membership. Balint tended to favour the former.

A crucial question was whether and when the *transference* to the leader should be confronted or interpreted. In general Balint saw little point in drawing the GPs' attention to their relationship with himself unless it was very clearly a repetition of a feature of the case that had been presented; for example, if the group had been made to feel desperate by the story the doctor had told and was pressing Balint very hard to work some sort of magic, he might remark that it was very hard to bear being made to feel impotent. This may be seen as a fairly modest and oblique interpretation of the transference, but it has the virtue of not inviting further exploration of it in the here-and-now and was probably quite intelligible to this band of hard-pressed doctors. He did, however, constantly keep a close eye on how the group was seeing him or using him in case an interpretation of it, made only to himself, might alert him to an unobserved feature of the case to which he could then draw attention. Some colleagues thought that when such a shaft of light came mysteriously out of the blue from the leader, the GPs were liable to be so impressed that an underlying worshipful dependence was thereby encouraged. But Balint was not much impressed by this argument.

It quite often happened that various features of the doctor–patient relationship presented by one of the GPs reverberated in the group and became reproduced in the way members treated one another and the leader. This Balint considered 'public property' and so it could be confronted and interpreted freely. Indeed, as groups became more experienced, a GP was often the first to initiate this kind of understanding. There was nevertheless a limit to be set on how far interpretation could be carried in relation to a GP's behaviour. In so far as their behaviour impinged on and was revealed in their reported work with patients, Balint felt that by the GPs' having joined the group in the first place they had given permission for it to be scrutinized and interpreted. But in so far as this behaviour was quite evidently a pervasive tendency of their personality, a more far-reaching interpretation had not been legitimated. Balint was quite clear about this rule, and although it is a good deal easier to state than to follow, he very rarely broke it – except, perhaps, when he had become exasperated by the way the group's work was being obstructed by the behaviour.

So much for the method he developed. Of course, he was not the paragon of analytic virtues suggested above and often found himself lost or up a blind alley or worse. But he was able to learn from most of his mistakes, often with difficulty, and what remained in the experience of those who worked alongside him was his reliance on the principles of psychoanalysis.

But what of the content of the work he did in these groups? Implicit in his approach, never verbalized in the group but often discussed in the staff seminar, was a recognition that the work to be done was in the area of the *Oedipus complex*: the inhibitory influence of archaic authority figures in their minds on what the GPs could allow themselves to know and then to make use of. An encroachment by the GP onto the territory of the supposed expert and the revelation that the latter was no more than flesh and blood not only robbed the GP of a comfortable illusion but also stirred anxieties in him or her associated with parricide and hubris. It was, however, only by traversing this rocky path that GPs could free themselves of the thraldom of their 'elders and betters' and get down to using their own observations and judgement in their experience of general practice, assisted, of course, by their peers in the group. It became evident to the GP that a capacity to accept some things that were said and to reject others on the basis of their own experience was their most valuable asset. It seemed that for some GPs their medical training had been so overwhelming that their capacity for *reality-testing* had been seriously impaired, in which case it was the job of the group to reawaken their curiosity and to strengthen such capacity for reality-testing as they had. This was further reinforced by Balint's insistence that whenever possible follow-up contacts with patients were reported to the group. By this means the convivial excitement of making new discoveries together was harnessed to the demands of professional practice, and limits were set to the growth of self-congratulatory illusions. In the staff seminar it was the formulation of the Oedipus complex that threw most light on the trials and tribulations of trying to lead a so-called 'Balint Group'.

As the GPs began to grasp that certain aspects of their relationships with their patients were products of the *repetition compulsion* in both their patients and themselves, so their interest in their professional work deepened and the power of *psychic reality* became apparent to them by implication. These, however, were never discussed as such, and the vocabulary that became current was more Sullivanian and interpersonal than intrapsychic: the concepts of *internal objects* or part-objects, for example, were never heard of, though they might well have been used in the staff seminar during their technical discussions.

In the course of their work there were the inevitable spells of excitement and despondency. When they were low spirited and ruminative the GPs doubtless stayed fairly quiet with their patients; but when in a spell of excitement they were certainly inclined to be wild and intrusive with them. The accusation that the groups produced half-trained *wild psychotherapists* could not be denied altogether. A fearfully evangelic spirit can follow the dawning of an insight that has long been held under.

Early in the training scheme, when Balint still thought it to be feasible for GPs to develop a way of working in the style of professional psychotherapists, the GPs who were inclined to embark on long interviews of face-to-face, confrontational and interpretative psychotherapy were offered supervision. But this never proved satisfactory and for a number of reasons fell away. By degrees the GPs developed a whole range of uses for the insights they were now open to: kindly tolerance, humorous acceptance, intermittent reflection of the patient to himself, deliberate choice of the right moment for a confrontation, occasional interpretative forays, and so forth. But in the process of each GP finding out what suited his or her attributes best experimentation was inevitable with occasional deplorable excesses; namely, *acting-out.*

The psychoanalytically trained leader was naturally made to feel extremely uncomfortable by what sometimes appeared to be going on in the doctor's surgery or in their patient's home. With his professional dignity offended he often forgot that pain and suffering are not always caused by incautious interventions, but sometimes by keeping silent for fear of overstepping the mark: caution can be as damaging as foolhardiness but is less obvious and shaming. Nevertheless, the dilemma posed some important questions about the training process.

It was assumed that such an episode of ill-judged or intrusive behaviour was the result of the GP identifying with an image of a psychoanalyst inflated by his own excitement, caused by a flash of new understanding. Furthermore, it was assumed that this parody of an analyst was also intended as an attack upon him and a triumphing over him, all of which should be expected in the course of an Oedipal struggle. How then should the group leader respond to this situation: a professional misdemeanour that is also a step in a valuable process of development?

In psychoanalytic training the candidate's struggle with their internal authority figures now projected onto their analyst is the stuff of their analysis. In the setting of the candidate's analytic work with this patient, however, should there be any acting-out in this way it can be moderated in the session with the candidate's supervisor, who has a clear responsibility in this matter. Ideally, enough work would have been done in the candidate's own analysis to make such a leakage into clinical work unlikely; but circumstances are rarely ideal. In a training group of professionals, however, the leader is in a difficult position: if they intervene and try to put a stop to it, they inevitably play a confirmatory part in the doctor's unconscious phantasy of a battleground and cut short a possible developmental step; if they do nothing, they collude with the doctor in a situation that can be damaging to all concerned, including the public reputation of the whole training scheme; if they interpret the doctor's behaviour effectively in the light of the above dynamics, they risk becoming an even more exciting object in the doctor's inner world but are in a poor position to take up the consequences of having made the interpretation in the first place – that is, the reader has practised wild analysis himself.

Leaders differed in how they struggled with the appearance of wild analysis in their groups. Balint himself came to keep a very firm eye on the fact that the GPs were there to be helped with the work they were actually engaged in and were not to be drawn onto some ill-defined intermediate ground of imitative psychotherapy. As a result, when faced with some work that was becoming wild he would usually try to rouse the other GPs to react to what had been reported in the hope that it would reassert the culture of general practice. Alternatively, he would call for another case to be presented by some other doctor to bring the whole group down to earth again. He appreciated that it was only the GPs' reliance on their own professional judgement as to what was useful and what was not in the course of their very arduous work that would save them from some fanciful flirtations with psychoanalysis.

Certainly there are some advantages in the method used in psychoanalytic training: the candidate's own analysis is not distorted by his analyst's suddenly taking up a supervisory role, and the candidate's supervisor can be quite explicit in criticizing his clinical work when necessary. The supervisor has the authority to do this and the candidate can be quite clear about the difficulty. This situation reinforces the candidate's identification with psychoanalysis as demonstrated by the two analysts, which is quite appropriate for someone learning that particular skill. Incidentally, it may also contribute to some of the piety in the psychoanalytic movement with its cliques and schools. But for a GP such an identification would be disastrous. Using the Balint Method every effort was made to reinforce the GP's authority in what they did or didn't do so that they would adopt new ways learned in the group only to the extent that they themselves found them useful in the light of experience. The leader's aim was to offer a model that would facilitate this kind of development when internalized and would not impose a new and foreign set of standards: to be an addition to the ego rather than to the superego.

It must be said, however, that Balint only found his way through this gradually. He was himself an enthusiastic therapist with many ideas on how therapy might be conducted in less than a five-times-a-week analysis. Early in the training scheme this enthusiasm was unabated and stirred up a number of experiments that sometimes outstripped the GPs' sober professional judgements. He was an exciting and challenging person to be with, and it was this same quality that fired the project in the first place and that kept the research element in it alive. But he could learn from experience, and as the GPs found that the gains for them were substantial but very varied and usually bore little resemblance to formal psychotherapy, he modified his aims.

The days when the accusation of encouraging wild or half-baked psychotherapy had some validity were the early ones before Balint had learned his lesson and before discussions among the leaders had clarified some of the technical factors that had encouraged it. In the early days a good deal of alarm and criticism was stirred up within the psychoanalytic fraternity, some of it with good reason. But by degrees and with difficulty the staff were also able to adapt their psychoanalytic fervour to the realities of a GP's life. Development was not the prerogative of the GPs alone.

A disturbance of the GP's professional competence less vivid or notable than 'wild analysis' was a transient loss of some of their older well-tried responses to their patients' needs. Though as a result of the group's work the GP might ultimately regain these responses in modified forms and with more discretion as to their uses, for a while they seemed to be ousted by a tendency to be compulsively passive listeners. For a while one would hear very little of the doctors being firm with their patients, or masterful, or even harsh, responses that might have been urgently called for, in fact. As the leaders themselves began to feel more at home in the unfamiliar setting of a GP group they were able to be firmer in their management of their work in it: to stop a slide into therapy, to stop a participant taking up so much time as to suggest that 'no other patients were waiting', to raise a humdrum issue when the discussion was becoming rarefied or academic, and so on – even to eject a member whose obstructive behaviour seemed obdurate and had become too much for the leader to bear. A leader who lost sight of his task in the group must have done little to help the GPs to stick to the realities of their own work, the conditions of general practice and the particularities of their personalities, so that although the changes wrought in the GP's personality were bound to entail some emotional turmoil, the leader's technique could play an important part in mitigating its interference with the GP's professional competence. Unlike analysis, this did not depend primarily on framing an apposite interpretation except in so far as, given to himself, it might guide the leader's hand as to what to do next.

It is hard for many analysts to understand what the benefit for medical practice might be from Balint's work if it is not some oblique teaching of formal psychotherapy, which it most emphatically is not. During and since his time many articles have been written describing uses that busy GPs have been able to make of it – for example, E. Balint and J. Norell (1973) and Elder and Samuel (1987). As an example among many, an account by one GP is given in Chapter 10. Likewise his work has been carried forward in many ways and in many settings, sometimes, it must be said, in ways that have strayed so far from the Balint Method described here as to be likely to make him turn in his grave – usually by falling into a mode of teaching, either teaching good general practice or teaching erudite psychopathology.

Finally, what are we to make of the eponymous legacy: the Balint Method, Balint Groups, the Balint Society? Certainly these are useful shorthand terms. But do they not also mean that his contribution has not been fully understood and assimilated? If it had been, we would be content with operational and technical terms to refer to it. As it is, some mystery remains hidden in the use of his name, and, if we are not careful, by using it we let ourselves off from the task he set himself and pursued in such a sincere and robust way. There is always the questionable delight of having one's mind taken by storm and of embalming him in it.

10

Moments of change

ANDREW ELDER

The context of our study was the day-to-day world of general practice. Patients coming and going, bringing the widest imaginable variety of symptoms and troubles, pains and anxieties, difficulties in relationships and illnesses. It is a world of powerful feelings, some arising from expectations before even the first meeting, and others that develop between the doctor and patient over time. There is a mass of physical symptoms, some of which the doctor must relieve, others he must learn to leave alone, and yet others he must respond to, yet not cure, as though courageously failing on repeated occasions, without losing heart and rejecting the patient. There are illnesses that need the doctor's attention, and others which protect their owners from something worse, that need the doctor's understanding. It is a world where the doctor is frequently in the dark, getting glimpses of his or her patients from time to time, being careful not to find out too much, being content to find the right distance for the patient and the doctor; sometimes needing to take the initiative, at others needing to be more restrained, waiting patiently for the developing pattern of the doctor–patient relationship to emerge.

There is a steady flow of patients in and out, but the doctor is a relatively fixed figure. He or she is available in a more or less constant fashion, and frequently works in the same community for most of a professional lifetime. But of course the doctor's own world is changing too. They have their own reactions to particular patients and particular problems. They have their own attitudes to illness, suffering, ageing and death, and their own strengths and limitations in human relationships just as their patients have. GPs who sit behind their desks hoping to make all their patients better will soon be exhausted and disillusioned. Doctors in general practice have to learn to live with their patients in a much more unchanging world than often both would wish. The frustration of this has to be borne, just as uncertainty also has to be, in order to allow other possible changes to occur.

One of the questions for our study was to what extent do these two worlds – the doctor's and the patient's – meet in moments of understanding between the two? Most of the time such contact is not sought. The day-to-day business of general practice is carried on according to the doctor's style of working and the problems of their patients. Sometimes, however, there is a greater need for understanding. The patient may be disclosing important aspects of themselves and the difficulties they are experiencing, in the way that they bring their symptoms to the doctor. Can the doctor now tune in sufficiently to form a useful relationship with the patient?

It is part of a general practitioner's job to be accessible to their patients. Much emphasis is also laid nowadays on a general style of personal accessibility in consulting technique. The doctor should be relaxed and welcoming, allowing the patient to talk and ask questions. Often on training schemes such approaches are taught with the help of video-tape recordings of consultations. A consulting style can be temporarily modified by this sort of behavioural feedback, but it may not fit comfortably with the doctor's personality. What of the doctor's more personal world? The 'video' is also needed in the doctor's head, as a third eye, monitoring not only the doctor's behaviour but his or her reactions and feelings in response to the patient as well. This can enable the doctor to make freer and fuller use of their own personality with patients – a freeing from within their range of possibilities as opposed to an imitative addition from without.

Patients, then, have their 'presentation' and doctors have their professional 'style' and 'technique'. How much of a real communication can there be? How much of the patient's world can the doctor appreciate? And if, for a moment, there is a contact, how does it affect the relationship afterwards? What changes in whom? These are difficult questions to study in any setting. In general practice they are doubly so because of the varied and transitory nature of the contacts. And yet probably there is no other setting with such a ferment and range of human activity within it.

In *Six Minutes for the Patient* (E. Balint and J. Norrel 1973) a new technique was described in which

> the doctor is freed from the primary task of trying to discover *why* the patient talks, thinks, feels and behaves in the way he does . . .; the doctor's task is primarily to observe a very small sample of *how* the patient talks, thinks and behaves and *why* this causes him pain . . . what really makes him want the doctor's attention.

> (Enid Balint)

After working along these lines, the authors of the book described the result of their study as the 'flash' technique. A 'flash' occurred when the doctor and patient suddenly 'saw' the significance of their work together.

The doctor has to allow himself the discomfort of abandoning his own ideas of what should be happening and 'tune in' to the patient's distress. Often the flash concerns the relationship between doctor and patient, but even if it does not, the relationship is changed by the flash.

The emphasis of this technique doesn't lie in discovering secrets, or relating past to present. It leaves the initiative with the patient and draws the maximum strength from the natural time-scale of general practice: brief contacts within a long-term context. 'The therapy, we think, lies in the peculiar intense flash of understanding between the doctor and patient in a setting where an ongoing contact is possible, where neither the doctor nor the patient gives up his self-esteem' (Enid Balint).

In our group we were interested to examine how the insights and techniques of the earlier work were being applied ten years later. We chose to base our work on a study of those interviews which seemed to contain a sudden change in the relationship between the doctor and the patient. The doctors in the group brought along cases in which something had 'seemed to happen' or 'a change' had occurred, and these were then discussed.

There may be many moments in consultations when the doctor more or less successfully hears what the patient is communicating and tunes in. But occasionally, more significant interviews seem to occur, which contain moments when the doctor's whole view of the patient may change. This is a little like the beam from a lighthouse suddenly bringing to light a new shape; it may have always been there, but it is suddenly seen, illuminated for the first time, and once seen alters the subsequent memory of the landscape. We are not looking at moments which would be accompanied by any obvious behavioural change, but rather at something more intangible, a psychological event, occurring in either the patient, or the doctor, or between both; a pivotal point, around which a change in relationship occurs.

It is often the case that what is most easily measured is of least interest, and what is of most interest is very hard to measure. If we felt an important moment had occurred that changed things between a doctor and a patient, how could we demonstrate this? How could we define the change and relate it to the important moment? There were too many uncertainties to attempt validating our work by making and ascertaining the accuracy of predictions. Instead we felt our approach had to be that of the natural historian: to attempt honest descriptive work and hope that it would be found useful.

113

RALPH Y

One of the doctors reported a contact with a patient who in many senses might be thought 'a hopeless case'. She had seen him just two or three days previously and the interview turned out to last about twenty minutes.

He's a man called Mr Y, aged 63. Um, he's been with the practice for about four years and I know him to be a longstanding alcoholic who pops in and out of the liver unit at the local hospital, and I haven't had very many previous contacts with him but those that I have had have been somewhat discouraging in the sense that he's one of a number of patients who one feels is probably a somewhat unhelpable alcoholic. . . . He had had a recent brief admission with a bleeding gastric ulcer. . . . So he came in . . . said he's got a cough . . . . He wasn't in any way incapacitated, but obviously he had had a drink sometime that day and so really I was quite prepared to treat his cough and not do anything very much else. . . . I sort of did the ritual examination of his chest and was thinking that perhaps I had better give him an antibiotic. And for some reason I decided that perhaps, you know, one should once again talk about this drinking and . . . He said that in 1978, after he's been in the hospital and had really been pretty ill . . . there'd been some kind of group formed at the hospital which he's attended regularly for more than two years and during that time with that support he'd managed to keep off the booze but the group had packed up because the person who was running it had gone somewhere else and so . . . since then he didn't really know quite why he'd started again but he couldn't do without his bottle of Martini because the withdrawal symptoms he'd got were so bad . . . but he said he just feels as if he's strangled and can't breathe . . . knows that his days are numbered . . . I think he is, actually, is desperately wanting to stop but yet terribly frightened of this every night feeling that he is choking. . . . And, what he apparently does is he doesn't buy his bottle until the evening. He drinks three-quarters of it and then he drinks the other quarter in the morning. I mean, to get through the night and then to get started again in the morning . . . at some point I was beginning to feel more sympathetic to him and he was sort of warming up a bit and sort of being more communicative . . . he said I'm a homosexual and a psychologist had given him the name of a homosexual group in London . . . nothing to do with alcoholics, just as a kind of support group that he might get in touch with and he thought that that might be quite a good idea. So I agreed. . . . I asked him if he'd ever tried the AA and he said Yes, and he didn't care for it very much. . . . It seemed really that he was quite

114

prepared to be serious again about stopping drinking and I started trying to discuss with him the practicalities of it, whether he would be willing to go into the hospital again to be dried. . . . But he said that he couldn't possibly go into hospital at the moment because he is about to lose his present job. He's a storeman by trade. He's worked in a family firm for many years and the people who run the firm know him very well and presumably have put up with his problems over the years, but the firm is packing up and he has in fact got a job to go to, starting on Monday in a shop, and he said at 63 he obviously isn't going to get another offer of a job and this one has been engineered for him I think by his former employers and so he's very anxious to go to the job. As he gets bad withdrawal symptoms I thought well, if I could tide him over a few days with Heminevrin, which isn't a drug I'm very familiar with or very happy about using . . . he might be able to get through the next week or two. . . . I was hoping I was talking in terms of seeing him again on Monday or Tuesday to try and keep hold of him. . . . I referred back to what he said about this group and so I said I knew he hadn't any family and I said 'Do you have any friends or contacts?' and he said, well, the only sort of friends he's got are these people in the shop that he's been working for. And I said had . . . I asked him if he had any homosexual friends or contacts and he said no he hadn't and it was a bit hard. He was very lonely, obviously. And I asked him if he'd been in trouble with the police and he said only once and that was about fifteen years ago. . . . I sort of arranged that he would ring me up on Monday to tell me how he was and so on. And he was about to leave and then he reminded me gently that we'd forgotten about his cough which I was going to prescribe for. So I added an antibiotic for his chest. As he was going he said something about 'I seem to have taken up a lot of your time.' And it was actually twenty minutes. And he went off, looking quite cheerful and I felt quite cheerful about it at the end of the consultation as he went out I felt a bit hopeful about him. Um, but I don't know . . . I had after-thoughts.

This seems at first sight a fairly straightforward business. The doctor sees a patient and decides to perform what is asked of her and not enquire much further. Her first impression is that this man is something of a hopeless case. Her diagnosis might have been 'chest infection in a chronic alcoholic with poor prognosis'. However, as the doctor mentions later in the group discussion, she has 'recently been successful with another chap with a long history of drinking', and perhaps this, together with the feeling of warmth she notices in herself at one stage, is sufficient to prompt her into making a few enquiries and listening a bit as the patient explains how important it is for him to hold on to his new job. A feeling of sympathy is aroused and the doctor's conscience is stirred: 'Something he said to me, you know, I just felt that I couldn't deliberately shut my eyes to his enormous problem and just deal with his little problem.'

There is no dramatic change in the relationship here, and there does not seem to have been an important moment. The doctor's world and the patient's world do not seem particularly close, but there is a movement during the interview away from the original conception of a 'lonely homosexual alcoholic with liver failure' towards somebody of whom the doctor can say, 'He's not just an alcoholic, so that if he comes back still drinking, he's a person and I do care about him.' The patient most likely has had a lifelong experience of being rejected. He is not someone who would come expecting the doctor's individual attention and may well be rather ashamed or overwhelmed to receive it. One of the doctor's comments in the discussion was, 'This is a man who gets pushed off, isn't it? He wasn't bleeding too badly so they let him out again . . . you don't let people go when they're not bleeding *too badly*!' It is easy to imagine a busy doctor choosing to deal with such a case quickly in order to catch up on the morning surgery. The presenting doctor has not been shocked by this man, nor fired with too great a zeal for reforming him. She has not tried too hard to get him to give up alcohol or delved too much into his homosexuality. She has accepted him and tried to help in a way that any experienced general practitioner would have done.

As discussion of the case in the group developed there seemed to be general agreement that what the doctor had achieved with this patient was valuable: 'This is getting the atmosphere right so that you can engage with the patient in a working sort of way. Regardless of the fact that he may feel, oh my God, she's talking about the booze I had!'

At the same time there was a persistent doubt that ran through the discussion of this case. Was there another area of more intense contact between these two that never quite occurred? If so, was that nearer to what we were trying to study?

This other theme is opened in the group discussion by one doctor who remarks, 'I think that if you concentrate on trying to stop him drinking, you'll miss doing the really important work, the possible work, and I feel very gloomy about it.'

This possible work that came close to the surface but did not quite break into the open seemed to be associated with the patient's terror of the night, his feeling of suffocation. This was the direction in which strong and immediate feelings seemed to lie. 'I think he needs to share how just absolutely intolerable it is looking at the night, he can cope with the day when he is working. It's just that he obviously dare not go to sleep without his bottle.'

116

The patient, lonely and frightened, is nearing death. He has probably been frightened of darkness, the night-time and being alone, all his life. Could such a feeling be shared? What would have to happen in the doctor's mind to make such a sharing possible? Intellectual recognition that this was a likely aspect of the patient's experience would not be sufficient to spark a moment of real contact.

We often referred in our discussions to 'changing gear' and 'levels of engagement'. Perhaps we can see three or four possible 'gears' or 'levels' in this case.

Dr A sizes the situation pretty quickly and decides to give the minimum that is asked. He knows that he has made that choice and does not feel too badly about it. He recognizes that he cannot do everything for everybody, and keeps his head down when the outlook doesn't look too promising. The doctor in the case had probably been a Dr A on the first few occasions of seeing this patient.

Dr B, however, might seize on this patient, regarding the chest infection as the patient's 'ticket of entry' and his alcoholism, or possibly even his homosexuality, as the 'real problem', something general practititioners should be on the look-out for and 'manage'. He would take various 'appropriate' steps – withdrawal from alcohol first, then social support, homosexual counselling and so on: textbook management without much regard for the person. Dr B would be a little like a parent who, facing the patient frightened at night, clutching on to his bottle, reacts by trying to take it away, saying, 'That'll do you no good. You had better give it up.'

Dr C is different. He sees an unhappy man, feels some sympathy for his condition, and allows him time and human breathing space. He paves the way for making himself a useful doctor for this patient in the future. The parental voice in Dr C is saying, 'I can see you're in a mess and do need your alcohol. I can accept that, and realize that it'd be more or less impossible for you to live any other way. It'd be nice if you could, but I'll be here if you can't. I'll encourage you if you do well and I won't be too accusing and rejecting if you fail.' This seems close to the doctor's actual management.

The voice of Dr D is the echo in the group discussion. This time the doctor goes along with the patient as above, but also allows just enough of the patient's main communication, perhaps terror, into his own experience at that moment, to feel something of his own terror of death and being left alone. Such an experience may alter for some time the relationship be-tween the doctor and patient; with the doctor seeing the patient more vividly and responding to him from a richer perspective, while the patient perhaps also experiences the doctor in a different light. Later in the discussion one of the doctors says, 'But supposing he relapses and he gets to work a bit blotto, crashes the van and gets the boot. I mean, or whatever, and then slides into alcohol. He's been seen for one moment as a real person himself in trouble and heard. I think that would make the work valid, regardless.'

Such moments cannot be manufactured or prescribed, but they seem more likely to occur when thoughts of management, or 'changing things for the better' are furthest from the doctor's mind.

This case is only an example, selected for the purpose of description. It is a fraction of a doctor's work, in one morning, held under scrutiny. There was much discussion of what aims would be appropriate for such a case anyway. Every doctor would have done differently. Perhaps one approach to this is to say that the doctor must be free enough at the time of the consultation to review the various possibilities in his mind.

It is clear from the follow-up reports that the doctor did become someone to whom this lonely and unhappy man could turn for help. He did get into trouble with the new job and began drinking heavily, but came to the doctor earlier than he might have done, and was admitted for 'drying out'. There was more and more emphasis on his 'drinking problem'. He came often and had been seen twenty-seven times in a year at the last follow-up report. The relationship seemed to be settling into the kind doctor and the unfortunate man. In one follow-up report there is mention of the patient's dread of being found in a coma, taken for dead and buried alive.

None of the doctors who were in the group are trained psychotherapists and few have had experience of personal therapy or analysis. They were, however, all experienced in the use of such psychotherapeutic skills as are commonly used in general practice. We were not concerned with describing the effects of these skills themselves. They are part of the mature doctor's technical equipment, along with his stethoscope, ophthalmoscope and pharmacopoeia. We were more interested in studying the tuning of the doctor's whole response to the patient. It often needs a quite unusual occurrence, a jolt, for the doctor to change. In most cases the doctor had tried all his usual tricks and exhausted his bag of skills. These were doomed because they all lay within the restrictions of the present relationship between the doctor and patient. A change was needed to bring the two into greater contact with each other. The doctor may be working more or less effectively within the focus of his present understanding, and this may include his use of various psychological skills which help the relationship along. But in the work we are trying to describe, the change that occurs is a sudden enlargement of this focus itself. The whole voltage of his understanding goes up. It is a sudden change of the context, rather than the content of the doctor–patient relationship, that is important.

STUART M

The doctor had known Mr M for about four years before discussing the case in the group and had usually found him a rather exasperating patient. He described his previous relationship with him in the following way: 'Irritating and unexpressive – looks incredulous and superior. I had usually felt like "shaking" him.' He had never used this feeling, and instead had treated him with exaggerated caution – 'kid gloves'. He reported two interviews, almost a month apart, in which the usual pattern of their relationship seemed to change.

> He is a tall, rather expressionless, very superior sort of thin chap . . .
> who was a student when I first came across him – I should think in
> about 1975 when he was due to take some exams . . . presented a lot
> of escalating anxiety things before his exams and pulled out of them.
> I think this happened at least two or three times; very similar patterns,
> he came with insomnia and restlessness and lots of sort of symptoms
> linked with anxiety which was focused entirely on his forthcoming
> exams.

The doctor never felt effective at helping him with this and used to see him increasingly frequently as his exams approached, and ended up prescribing a different and stronger tranquillizer, until Mr M would suddenly with-draw, go home, and things would calm down a bit until the following year. After this cycle recurred two or three times, the doctor felt desperate himself and referred the patient to a counsellor who worked in his health centre.

> She saw him in fact weekly for a year and we used to discuss him from
> time to time. . . . Exactly the same cycle recurred . . . he used the
> sessions only as a mechanism to do with exam passing . . . he left
> college and never got a degree. He took a temporary job as a driver
> at a local firm, and is still there, two years later.

The doctor had later seen him when he had been found to have iritis and the firm wouldn't employ him until it was fully investigated and treated. He had become a frequent attender with anxiety symptoms. It was against this background of the doctor feeling stuck with this patient that he began his report of the more recent interviews.

> He started with various physical symptoms, as though he'd never seen
> me much before. . . . Incredibly boring and very, very detailed,
> terribly distant, a very controlled sort of aggression about doctors and
> things . . . a long story, with many minute physical symptoms: he had
> tingling sensations and had gone to the occupational health service

who had said it was anxiety, and then gone to casualty and they'd given him some Valium which he chucked across my desk in a very disparaging way . . . then he'd gone – and really he knows me well, up to his parents and seen their doctor who had given him some Ativan and again the same sort of inadequate transaction in his view . . . was described.

The doctor clearly thinks that the patient should not be rejecting his efforts like this, and should have responded sooner to his therapeutic endeavours, but the patient feels differently. He feels helpless and unhelped – and this feeling he successfully passes on to the doctor, who now describes mounting fury.

I felt really furious with him and actually gave him . . . a good sort of bashing, though in a rather, a sort of covert way. I mean, I said how difficult he found it to trust anyone and how awful it must feel to him to have such useless doctors who couldn't help him and it must leave him feeling very helpless. . . . He looked very stunned and said he wasn't worried about anything. Had no worries. I then said that perhaps it wouldn't be a bad thing if he did . . . it wouldn't be such a disaster . . . instead of floating above it all the time. . . . And he looked pretty stunned about that and I felt fairly bad after it . . . and followed up saying . . . we must take your symptoms seriously and went through a careful physical examination . . . it was a full half-hour.

There was a gap of a month before the patient consulted the doctor again. The interview had stayed alive in the doctor's mind and it seems in the patient's too, as he had twice come to the surgery and seen different doctors, who both passed on messages to the doctor about the patient. It seemed as though he had needed to keep away but also to let the doctor know that he was still around. The patient started by telling the doctor of his recent appointments and his symptoms. The doctor commented that it was like exam-time again, but this time there were no exams. The patient responded by saying he was a bit worried about work and still being there, and had had a bit of trouble with his landlady. He liked the firm, finding the work enjoyable, 'the people are fun – though my parents are worried, they say ah, well, if you like it'.

I asked him whether his parents were always so understanding with him . . . so tolerant. . . . He looked at me rather surprised and said Yes, well, of course. . . . He looked down and talked for a bit and then said, yes, maybe what I do need is a bit of a kick up the backside.

This was the click back to the last interview and quite a sudden clue to the relationship.

I said . . . that's very much what I'd felt I'd given him last time and that maybe he could survive a good kick now and then. I asked him why his father hadn't ever given him one? . . . Maybe he felt intimidated, or inhibited, or something.

The doctor was conscious of his own rather cautious and inhibited handling of the patient. He remarked to the patient that he had often felt rather intimidated by him and perhaps the patient had more power over things than he realized. This produced a definite reaction in the patient, quite unlike anything he had shown of himself before.

. . . and this idea that he had been intimidating or that he was powerful shook him absolutely and then he sort of laughed and it was the first time I had seen this man really show some feelings. And he couldn't get over it. He was absolutely stunned. . . . You know, this power business. And he said, 'What?! Me?! Powerful? . . . intimidating? . . . absolutely not . . . and then he said something about how his parents had treated them all differently, there being four children. . . . It just left him obviously with some sort of new idea about himself . . . and that was that interview.

What seems to have happened here? All the doctor's endeavours to change, reform or cure the patient, whether by prescription, referral or trying to understand his background, have come to nothing. The patient remains firmly aloof. He brings along his mounting anxiety through symptoms and, as though detached from them in a rather superior way, gives them to the doctor to do something with. He then watches with disdain while the doctor, who seems to fall for this surprisingly readily, works away with mounting exasperation, trying everything he knows, and in so doing experiences more and more of the patient's helpless anxiety. Eventually he cannot stand it any longer. There is an abrupt reversal and sudden switching of the see-saw they have been on, with the doctor suddenly releasing his feelings through sarcasm. The patient crashes down. The doctor feels rather sorry and restores the balance a bit with a physical examination before the two part. Within this see-saw relationship there has been a powerful reversal fantasy. The patient has behaved as though he is on one side, appearing exaggeratedly humble and helpless, while seeing the doctor, on the other side, as powerful and mighty. This view is communicated with an irritating irony which seems to say that really the opposite is the truth; the doctor's efforts are laughable while the patient is above it all. The sudden release of feeling in the doctor was one kind of important moment but, more important, the echo was still heard a month later when the theme re-emerged. The doctor was sufficiently in tune this time. He was more watchful and less angry. The doctor, instead of anxiously playing along with the patient as he has done previously, admits that the patient has often made him feel rather intimidated and helpless. It is this sudden spoken thought of what the patient may have wished for some time that is too much for him. The brake is off. Pleasurable disbelief breaks out. Incredulity. There is an important moment shared. They are able to hold the see-saw for a while in a more even and realistic position. There is greater warmth and a greater area of exchange between the two.

We often discussed in the group the difference between a change in the doctor–patient relationship and a change in the patient's world outside. Clearly it is the latter that is usually the aim of a doctor's work. It is easier to observe changes in the relationship; through the atmosphere of the consultation, the doctor's feelings, the symptoms that the patient brings or the frequency of contact. We were always less certain about how these changes were reflected in whatever changed in the patient's general life. There were always other factors which could have influenced things. But maybe there is more connection than we often observe or admit. In this case there seems to have been a change in the doctor–patient relationship, but what sort of change? How long will it last? And will it help lead to any other changes in the patient's life?

The first follow-up interview occurred at the doctor's request, just a week later, prompted only by my request for a follow-up the week before. The patient reported a complete improvement of his symptoms. 'You asked me to come back – I feel 100 per cent.' He mentioned how much failing at college had hurt – and we talked a bit about what had been said in the previous interview – but my main feeling was of scraping around and that there was nothing more to do for the present. It was a short, satisfactory 'nothing more to be said', probably unnecessary interview. The next one happened about six weeks later on the patient's initiative and

> This time the patient came to get a prescription for more drops for his iritis and said everything continued to be fine and he had no idea what caused his previous pain . . . he put me on the spot with some medical questions which I answered a bit uneasily . . . and felt he was sort of playing the exaggerated patient, and me being sort of cautious, you know, just answering questions. . . . He said he had begun thinking a bit about changing his job . . . he'd made some steps in going to see a careers adviser. He said something about, I think, something to do with microphones, a radio, working with radio. . . . It turned out he does research for radio programmes . . . but not in front of a microphone, he said, in a very typical self-disparaging. . . . I wouldn't dream of doing that, a thing in the public eye, oh no, not me with a little laugh. . . . We talked a bit about his need to be self-disparaging and fear of failure. He left with irritating but typical

exaggerated respect, shutting my door, which frequently slams, over-carefully, leaving me feeling it was shut with irony rather than consideration. This left me feeling in terms of the sort of interaction we had, nothing much had changed.

The group felt more confident about this than the doctor, who rather irritated them with his pessimism.

. . . Because there is a change, isn't there? That he's dropped his symptoms . . .

. . . I'm a bit puzzled about your attitude. . . . You find him much too humble and this is . . . is a terrific change . . .

. . . I mean can we relate what happens to what happened in the previous interview? I don't know whether we can or not. But there was a good shaking up, wasn't there?

. . . He was in danger of getting an overdose from the doctor, I think.

. . . I think we're a bit fed up with . . . I mean he irritated you by asking about symptoms . . . he irritated you badly. . . . But this time you should have been jolly gratified, I would have thought. . . . I would have liked to examine this syndrome about GPs being quite incapable of seeing when they do something good. I mean, this is an example, isn't it . . .?

. . . Yes, but this is one where the patient changes but the doctor still doesn't like this guy very much . . .

There seems to be general agreement that some things have changed. The patient has let go of his symptoms and seems to be capable of a more open approach with the doctor. He discusses his feelings of disappointment and rejection after failing at college and his fear of failure which keeps him out of the limelight and underachieving. He seems less superior and distant. The doctor seems to belittle his efforts and rather grandiosely seems to expect something more. The group disagrees, thinking he ought to feel gratified.

The patient has continued to see the doctor on average every two months and, although the intensity of the reported interviews isn't repeated, a useful relationship for the patient seems to have developed. There seems to have been a period of increased intensity, through which the relationship has changed, before settling into a new pattern.

If there was such a movement towards greater intensity in the reported interviews between this doctor and Mr M we might ask what prevented such a change occurring long before. The ingredients seem to have been there. Why was the relationship held in this rigid and rather unsatisfactory mode for so long? What sometimes releases the doctor? Or, conversely, what holds him back? Like W.H. Auden's Miss Gee, it often seems that doctors have a 'harsh back-pedal brake' applied to themselves, keeping their patients firmly fixed, at a certain distance. The brake reins back the doctor's own feelings, to allow his daily work to proceed. It may often be the case that some strong personal feelings are evoked for the doctor by association with the patient's predicament. Intimacy and engagement of the doctor's feelings have their cost. The interview ends, the patient may take some thoughts away or allow feelings to surface later, but the doctor has to lose them for the time being and start again with the next patient. Something needs to occur that allows the doctor to relax this inner professional device and release a greater freedom to feel, and think and respond with his patient. This requires an effort of imagination and sufficient relaxation for him to be both experiencing and using his own emotional world at the time of the consultation.

The question of what initiates this change and how it affects the patient was often discussed.

HANNAH V

One doctor introduced a case by saying, 'Well, I've got a sort of a one . . . in the sense that I've changed my view of the patient. I'm not sure if the patient's view of herself has in any way become different.'

Well, she's a lady of 71 . . . one of those people who came to this country from Germany in the 1930s . . . her name is Hannah. Her husband is her second husband. She's got a couple of kids by her first husband. I don't know what happened to that. It's also his second marriage. And he's about seven or eight years younger than she is. He's a travel agent and they've both been patients of mine for oh, eight, ten, fifteen years, something like that. And in that time she has had two hip replacements for osteoarthritis. I've had some medical dealing with her. And then last year, she became depressed and I treated her with good, sound, honest, decent pills [laughs] and, naturally, because she was properly treated she got better. . . . Her husband as I mentioned is younger than she is. . . . I know the son. I don't know the daughter who is older. When I first came into contact with this family some years ago, the son was living at home and I remember that he was a kind of 'yuk', who used to get venereal disease . . . and expect me to forget about that and organize it for him to be attended to. I mean, he really did get up my nose, yuk . . . to my astonishment he got married and is a respectable citizen. . . . Anyway, she came back to see me just before I went away on holiday, feeling depressed, having disturbed sleep, and being upset in the mornings and feeling better as the day wore on. Could she have some more of the whatever-it-was? So I gave her some and saw her after a couple of weeks just before I went away and arranged that she would see my partner when I was gone and scaled up the dose of drugs. So she got a bit better and came to see me when I got home again. . . . I have this image of her as a lady who has some physical disability. She's got this osteoarthritis that she'd had and she takes medicine for that. And she has pills for her depression. And when I was going on this holiday we discussed holidays . . . the family are in the travel agency business . . . had a sort of chatting, sort of friendly relationship. . . . This time she came she had seen my partner when I was away and she was glad to see me back and she was actually feeling terrible and it was awful. Could she perhaps try not the pills she was having, but the ones she'd had before? I just sort of didn't say very much and said, 'Well, you know, if things are bad, tell me why.' And all of a sudden she said, 'Well, you won't tell anyone.' Then it came out that her husband was having an affair with somebody at work, his secretary or something . . . and she feels that she is . . . it's natural that he should behave like this because she's so much older than he is. He is 64 only and they haven't had any sexual relations for some time . . . and why shouldn't he feel that way . . . and yet she feels it's not fair. And then I said something about 'it must feel very bad to come to this'. And she said, 'What?' And I realized for the very first time that she has a deaf aid. I suddenly saw her as an old woman with her whole life disappearing and it was something that I just hadn't seen at all. I had grown used to this patient and suddenly there she was, a lonely, desperate, deaf, deprived woman whose husband was deserting her and the children had left home. And all I could see suddenly was her disabilities and her future, or non-future. I suddenly sort of got hit by this tremendous sort of, oh! terrible feeling and guilt that I'd missed it all before. I don't know whether my feeling about her got across the deaf aid barrier, or what. I don't know what happened. But I do know that it suddenly hit me.

In the doctor's description there seems to be a friendly and rather conscientious aspect to the relationship. He chats about holidays and he carefully arranges for his partner to see the patient while he is away. There is also a feeling that he has held her somewhat at arm's length, perhaps not liking to come into too close contact with her misery, or maybe the memory of her 'awful' son is still active somewhere in his mind as a warning. He does not seem to have been able to let her talk to him before. They have had a 'decent' relationship but a rather distant one. There is a detached irony in some of the description – 'and, naturally, because she was properly treated she got better'. Only a little later on, we are suddenly hit with an awful vision of how this patient is feeling. Rejected and despairing. The doctor is stunned. He suddenly sees her as 'a lonely, desperate, deaf, deprived woman' whose husband is deserting her and whose children have left home. He is shocked. He concludes the interview but was probably hardly able to think after the impact of the important moment.

> I've been put off this family because of my feelings about the son. And I have had some sympathy with her in her physical disability.

> She had been hiding it up to now . . . there was something in her that didn't want to give you this . . . picture, possibly.

> Because she was sort of holding herself in and keeping alert and holding herself together, as well as possibly while you were away, and when you got back, she feels oh, hell, I'll show you what I'm really like.

> Is there a generation gap . . . the difference . . . that you were suddenly impressed with the age gap between you?

> For a long time you think of somebody as more or less your age, even if there is a twenty-year gap. And suddenly they move into a different generation.

> It was this sudden falling-apart thing. And also seeing her desperation. I had seen her as a pill-depressed patient, I suppose . . . and then all of a sudden, I saw genuine, total despair.

> I mean this is the sad thing that you weren't letting her talk to you before. This woman has had various replacements and has been growing old and she's been satisfied with the pills, and you've been satisfied with them and suddenly neither of you are. And I wonder what else has changed because she hasn't been letting her husband make love, but she tells you straight off. She's never mentioned this before. So what I am asking myself is 'Why did she suddenly tell you? Why not before? Why now?'

The patient seems to have had the habit of behaving well for the doctor in rather the same way as she makes herself younger for her husband. We know that often she finds herself to blame when other people reject her. 'It's natural that he should behave like this, because I'm so much older. . . . It's reasonable.' But when she comes for this interview her feeing of unfairness is closer to the surface than usual. She tells the doctor of her husband's interest in another woman and that she's been feeling awful and is glad to have the doctor back. It seems that the doctor's absence on top of what she is feeling anyway was too much. She can bear it no longer.

Up to this moment, the doctor seems to have been cruising in quite a relaxed fashion. He responds as he might often in a similar situation, by inviting the patient to tell him why she is feeling terrible, and then voices his reaction to what she says, 'It must feel very bad to come to this.' His remark, intended with empathy, only strikes a deafened 'What?' It is then that the true impact of her situation, and his reaction to it, hits him. The brake he has applied in his previous dealings with the patient is a little looser this time, and he allows enough of the patient's experience into his own to produce sudden change. It is as though the doctor has had an image of this patient that he has not wanted to see change and which she may have preferred him to have of herself. Suddenly it isn't sufficient for either of them. A further aspect of the reality of their relationship breaks through.

In this case there has been a dramatic change in the doctor's perception. But what effect, if any, does this have on the patient? Or on their relationship together?

> What's interesting is that the important moment was the doctor's shock, not the patient telling you about her miseries although it's quite important. . . . So what is the effect of the doctor's shock on the patient . . . it seems to me that this really is the question.

> This could happen with any patient. You think they are horrible but suddenly you see them differently and you do this visually . . . this is what we're talking about all the time.

> But do we assume that it's got to be a mutual thing for it to be effective? That's the question.

> This is why I brought it up . . . it seems to me that there's quite a real situation where she may have perceived absolutely nothing, and yet I'm quite certain that the way I will see her in the future will be different.'

What does the patient notice? As one doctor asked, 'Well, if she were in the seminar, what do you think she would be saying to her group?'
She returns to see the doctor a month later and is very depressed.

> She came back actually in October and she came in to say she wouldn't be seeing me for a month because she and her husband were going on safari – he's a travel agent and does tours for people and this, as it were, is an off-season inspection of the goods they are selling next year – so she's going to Africa on safari with him. And she wanted to talk to me first. Um, and she told me that she was depressed and afraid the pills I have given her were quite useless, that they were going on a safari and she was terrified that she was going

to spoil it. What had happened was that her husband and his girlfriend had decided that it was ridiculous and that they must break it off and he was now being very careful and good with her and she was scared that she was going to wreck the prospect of remaking their relationship on the holiday, because she was so down and awful. And she said that it was terrible the . . . if it really was the affair of his life, it was awful that she should ruin it for him, but on the other hand when they originally got engaged, because of their age differences, she pointed out that perhaps they shouldn't. Tears came into her eyes as she recalled how he had persuaded her after a long interval that they ought to live together and get married and . . . Since the girlfriend has been shed, she said that it's very difficult. He does everything right but he doesn't even want to touch her. He won't even kiss her and they certainly have no sex. I previously thought that sex had finished, but I am wrong; that apparently once the hip surgery and so forth had been dealt with, they had resumed normal marital relationships until this affair cropped up. But he isn't considerate at all . . . he does everything right, but it's not genuine. It's not real. And he has to force himself to do the right thing. And she feels how phoney it is and she says 'How can I . . . an old woman like me . . . cope with trying to remake a love affair with him? I love him still, but he doesn't love me and it's terrible. I don't know how I can cope.' So I said, 'You must be very cross with him for letting you down like this?' And she said: 'I am not cross with him. It's me, I'm a nuisance. How can I blame him for falling in love with a younger woman?' I felt very strongly the feeling that the insight that I had had was entirely legitimate about this interview. That it was . . . if you like, my insight didn't coincide in time with hers. She had had that kind of insight when she discovered about the affair and I picked it up and it was right. So what we were talking about wasn't the angry feelings that she has, but her desperation at falling apart and, um, she said: 'He tries to. . . . He's not considerate, he watches television and just tunes it to football.' Um . . . and she said she can't even tell him. 'I can't tell you how I feel, I lose the words.' 'What do you mean?' Well, she has a thick German accent. She said: 'I can't remember the words in English and I can't even remember them in German.' And we agreed that she comes and sees me when she comes back from this tour and she's gone off with considerable trepidation as to how the relationship is going to work.

This follow-up interview seems to confirm some of the seminar's views. The patient shows herself to be more obviously depressed with the doctor this time. There is less politeness and, instead of pretending that the doctor's pills have helped, she straightaway tells him they are useless. She is feeling miserable, but is too depressed to be angry and instead blames herself – 'It's me, I'm a nuisance'. She fears she will spoil things. The awfulness of the vision is verbalized this time. The doctor has steadied his balance. The patient's view isn't changed, but she has a doctor who has adjusted his hearing aid. Whereas previously the doctor–patient relationship seemed to mirror some of the difficulties with her husband, the doctor was polite but distant, not really wanting to 'touch' the patient, and she seemed to hold herself in for the doctor, for fear of spoiling things; now they do so less. The patient seems more confident of not being rejected, and the doctor can allow himself to listen better to her deeper and more unhappy feelings.

The doctor says:

> I don't feel as desperate this time as I did last time. Last time I felt completely paralysed by it. This time I felt I did quite real . . . work . . . I think that previously . . . I've been the doctor who dishes up the pills and is ever so kind from time to time, in brief. I think that I predict that we'll talk quite genuinely about feelings and about her relationship with her husband, and that my role will be supporting her through her depressive experience and, in a sense, valuing her as a real person rather than as a sort of degenerate wreck.

The patient has had a certain view of herself and the doctor has now tuned into it.

It seems likely from this case that the patient will be able to be different with her doctor in future and the doctor will 'feel' different to her. The doctor's matrix of assumptions about her has changed. A new insight may be produced by this sort of experience, but the 'giving' of insight isn't its purpose. It is more that a relationship is slowly built in such a way that the contact is a more real one, fuller, closer to the truth at the time. It enables the patient to experience himself more fully as a result. This may help to bring about a 'change' in the patient, but if so, it is almost incidental.

Michael Balint:
a select bibliography

1925   'Perversion or a Hysterical Symptom?', in *Problems of Human Pleasure and Behaviour: Classic Essays in Humanistic Psychiatry*, New York: Liveright, 1956, pp. 182–7. (Translation from Hungarian of a paper given in Berlin, 1923.)

1927   'I.P. Pavlov', in *Problems of Human Pleasure and Behaviour: Classic Essays in Humanistic Psychiatry*, New York: Liveright, 1956.

1932   'Psychosexual Parallels to the Fundamental Law of Biogenetics', in *Primary Love and Psychoanalytic Technique*, London: Hogarth Press, 1952, pp. 11–41, and (2nd, rev. edn) London: Tavistock Publications, 1965, pp. 3–30. (Translation of paper originally published in German, *Imago*, 1930.)

1933a   'The Psychological Problems of Growing Old', in *Problems of Human Pleasure and Behaviour: Classic Essays in Humanistic Psychiatry*, New York: Liveright, 1956, pp. 69–85. (Translation from Hungarian of a paper given in 1933.)

1933b   'Two Notes on the Erotic Component of the Ego-instincts', in *Primary Love and Psychoanalytic Technique*, London: Hogarth Press, 1952, pp. 42–8, and (2nd, rev. edn) London: Tavistock Publications, 1965, pp. 31–6. (Translation of a paper originally published in German, *International Journal of Psycho-Analysis*, 1933.)

1933c   'Character Analysis and New Beginning', in *Primary Love and Psychoanalytic Technique*, London: Hogarth Press, 1952, pp. 159–73 and (2nd, rev. edn) London: Tavistock Publications, 1965, pp. 151–64. (Translation from Hungarian of a paper given in 1932.)

1933d   'On Transference of Emotions', in *Primary Love and Psychoanalytic Technique*, London: Hogarth Press, 1952.

1934a   'The Adolescent's Fight against Masturbation', in *Problems of Human Pleasure and Behaviour: Classic Essays in Humanistic Psychiatry*, New York: Liveright, 1956, pp. 49–68. (Translation of a paper originally published in German, *Zeitung Psychoanal. Pädagogik*, 1934.)

1934b   'Dr Sandor Ferenczi as a Psychoanalyst', *Indian Journal of Psychology* 9:19–27. Reprinted in *Problems of Human Pleasure and Behaviour: Classic Essays in Humanistic Psychiatry*, New York: Liveright, 1956, pp. 235–42.

1935a   'A Contribution on Fetishism', *International Journal of Psycho-Analysis* 16(4): 481–3. Reprinted in *Problems of Human Pleasure and Behaviour: Classic Essays in Humanistic Psychiatry*, New York: Liveright, 1956, pp. 171–3.

1935b   'Critical Notes on the Theory of the Pregenital Organizations of the Libido', in *Primary Love and Psychoanalytic Technique*, pp. 49–72, and *Problems of Human Pleasure and Behaviour: Classic Essays in Humanistic Psychiatry*, New York: Liveright, 1956, pp. 37–58.

1936a   'The Final Goal of Psychoanalytic Treatment', *International Journal of Psycho-Analysis* 17(2): 206–16. Reprinted in *Primary Love and Psychoanalytic Technique*, London: Hogarth Press, 1952, pp. 188–99, and (2nd, rev. edn) London: Tavistock Publications, 1965, pp. 178–88.

1936b   'Eros and Aphrodite', *International Journal of Psycho-Analysis* 19(2): 199–213. Reprinted in *Primary Love and Psychoanalytic Technique*, London: Hogarth Press, 1952, pp. 73–9, and (2nd, rev. edn) London: Tavistock Publications, 1965, pp. 59–73.

1937a   'A Contribution to the Psychology of Menstruation', *Psycho-Analytic Quarterly* 6: 346–52. Reprinted in *Problems of Human Pleasure and Behaviour: Classic Essays in Humanistic Psychiatry*, New York: Liveright, 1956, pp. 174–81 (enlarged version).

1937b   'Early Developmental States of the Ego: Primary Object-love', *International Journal of Psycho-Analysis* 30(4): 265–73. Reprinted in *Primary Love and Psychoanalytic Technique*, London: Hogarth Press, 1952, pp. 90–108 and (2nd, rev. edn) London: Tavistock Publications, 1965, pp. 74–90.

1939a   (with Alice Balint) 'On Transference and Counter-transference', *International Journal of Psycho-Analysis* 20(3–4): 223–30. Reprinted in *Primary Love and Psychoanalytic Technique*, London: Hogarth Press, 1952, pp. 213–20, and (2nd, rev. edn), London: Tavistock Publications, 1965, pp. 201–8.

1939b   'Ego Strength and Education', *Psycho-Analytic Quarterly* 11(1): 87–95. Reprinted in *Primary Love and Psychoanalytic Technique*, London: Hogarth Press, 1952, pp. 200–12, and (2nd, rev. edn) London: Tavistock Publications, 1965, pp. 189–200, with the title 'Strength of the Ego and its Education'. (In both editions the Table of Contents lists this title as 'Strength of the Ego and Ego-pedagogy'.)

1942   'Reality Testing during Schizophrenic Hallucinations', *British Journal of Medical Psychology* 19(2): 201–14. Reprinted as 'Contributions to Reality Testing', in *Problems of Human Pleasure and Behaviour: Classic Essays in Humanistic Psychiatry*, New York: Liveright, 1956, pp. 153–70.

1948a   'On Genital Love', *International Journal of Psycho-Analysis* 29: 34–40. Reprinted in *Primary Love and Psychoanalytic Technique*, London: Hogarth Press, 1952, pp. 128–40, and (2nd, rev. edn) London: Tavistock Publications, 1965, pp. 109–20.

1948b   'On the Psychoanalytic Training System', *International Journal of Psycho-Analysis* 29(3): 163–73. Reprinted in *Primary Love and Psychoanalytic Technique* (2nd, rev. edn) London: Tavistock Publications, 1965, pp. 253–74.

1948c   'On Szondi's *Schicksalsanalyse* and *Triebdiagnostik*', *International Journal of*

Psycho-Analysis 29(4): 240–9. Reprinted in *Problems of Human Pleasure and Behaviour: Classic Essays in Humanistic Psychiatry*, New York: Liveright, 1956, pp. 261–80.

1949 'Dr Sandor Ferenczi, Obit. 1933', *International Journal of Psycho-Analysis* 30(4): 215–19. Reprinted in *Problems of Human Pleasure and Behaviour: Classic Essays in Humanistic Psychiatry*, London: Hogarth Press, 1957, pp. 243–50.

1950a 'Changing Therapeutical Aims and Techniques in Psychoanalysis', *International Journal of Psycho-Analysis* 31(3): 196–9. Reprinted in *Primary Love and Psychoanalytic Technique*, London: Hogarth Press, 1952, pp. 236–43, and (2nd, rev. edn) London: Tavistock Publications, 1965, pp. 223–9.

1950b 'On the Termination of Analysis', *International Journal of Psycho-Analysis* 31(3): 196–9. Reprinted in *Primary Love and Psychoanalytic Technique*, London: Hogarth Press, 1952, pp. 236–43, and (2nd, rev. edn) London: Tavistock Publications, 1965, pp. 223–9.

1951a 'The Problem of Discipline', *New Era* 2: 104–10. Enlarged version in *Problems of Human Pleasure and Behaviour: Classic Essays in Humanistic Psychiatry*, London: Hogarth Press, 1957, pp. 34–48.

1951b 'On Punishing Offenders', in G.B. Wilbur and W. Muensterberger (eds) *Psychoanalysis and Culture*, Reprinted in *Problems of Human Pleasure and Behaviour: Classic Essays in Humanistic Psychiatry*, New York: Liveright, 1956, pp. 86–116.

1952a *Primary Love and Psychoanalytic Technique*, London: Hogarth Press, *International Journal of Psycho-Analysis* Library.

1952b 'New Beginning and the Paranoid and the Depressive Syndromes', *International Journal of Psycho-Analysis* 33(2): 214–24. Reprinted in *Primary Love and Psychoanalytic Technique*, London: Hogarth Press, 1952, pp. 243–65 and (2nd, rev. edn) London: Tavistock Publications, 1965, pp. 230–49.

1952c 'On Love and Hate', *International Journal of Psycho-Analysis* 33(4): 355–62. Reprinted in *Primary Love and Psychoanalytic Technique*, London: Hogarth Press, 1952, pp. 141–56 and (2nd, rev. edn) London: Tavistock Publications, 1965, pp. 121–35.

1952d 'Notes on the Dissolution of Object-representation in Modern Art', *Journal of Aesthetics and Art Criticism* 10(4): 323–7. Reprinted in *Problems of Human Pleasure and Behaviour: Classic Essays in Humanistic Psychiatry*, New York: Liveright, 1956, pp. 117–24.

1952e (with S. Tarachow) 'General Concepts and Theory of Psychoanalytic Therapy', *Annual Survey of Psychoanalysis* 1: 227–40.

1954a 'Analytic Training and Training Analysis', *International Journal of Psycho-Analysis* 35(2): 157–62. Reprinted in *Primary Love and Psychoanalytic Technique* (2nd, rev. edn) London: Tavistock Publications, 1965, pp. 275–85.

1954b 'Geza Roheim: an Obituary', *International Journal of Psycho-Analysis* 35(4): 434–6. Reprinted in *Problems of Human Pleasure and Behaviour: Classic Essays in Humanistic Psychiatry*, New York: Liveright, 1956, pp. 256–60, under title 'Geza Roheim, 1891–1953'.

1954c '*The Life and Ideas of the Marquis de Sade* by G. Gover' (book review), *International Journal of Psycho-Analysis* 35(1): 78–83. Reprinted in *Problems of Human Pleasure and Behaviour: Classic Essays in Humanistic Psychiatry*, New York: Liveright, 1956, pp. 251–5.

1955a 'Notes on Parapsychology and Parapsychological Healing', *International Journal of Psycho-Analysis* 36(1): 31–5. Reprinted in *Problems of Human Pleasure and Behaviour: Classic Essays in Humanistic Psychiatry*, New York: Liveright, 1956, pp. 188–97.

1955b 'The Doctor, His Patient, and the Illness', *Lancet*: 683–8, 2 April 1955. Reprinted in *Problems of Human Pleasure and Behaviour: Classic Essays in Humanistic Psychiatry*, New York: Liveright, 1956, pp. 198–220.

1955c 'Friendly Expanses – Horrid Empty Spaces', *International Journal of Psycho-Analysis* 36(4–5): 225–41.

1956a *Problems of Human Pleasure and Behaviour: Classic Essays in Humanistic Psychiatry*, New York: Liveright, 1956.

1956b 'Pleasure, Object and Libido: Some Reflections on Fairbairn's Modifications of Psychoanalytic Theory', *British Journal of Medical Psychology* 29(2): 162–7. Reprinted in *Problems of Human Pleasure and Behaviour: Classic Essays in Humanistic Psychiatry*, New York: Liveright, 1956, pp. 281–91.

1956c 'Perversions and Genitality', in *Perversions, Psychodynamics and Psychotherapy*, New York: Random House, pp. 16–27. Reprinted in *Primary Love and Psychoanalytic Technique* (2nd, rev. edn), London: Tavistock Publications, 1965, pp. 136–44.

1956d 'Sex and Society', in *Problems of Human Pleasure and Behaviour: Classic Essays in Humanistic Psychiatry*, New York: Liveright, 1956.

1957a *The Doctor, His Patient and the Illness*, London: Pitman Medical Publishing.

1957b 'The Three Areas of the Mind: Theoretical Considerations', *International Journal of Psycho-Analysis* 39(5): 328–40. Reprinted in *The Basic Fault: Therapeutic Aspects of Regression*, London: Tavistock Publications, 1968, pp. 3–31.

1959a *Thrills and Regressions*, London: Hogarth Press.

1959b 'The Doctor's Responsibility', *Medical World* 92(6): 529–40. Reprinted in *Psychotherapeutic Techniques in Medicine* (with Enid Balint), London: Tavistock Publications, 1961, pp. 104–15.

1960a 'Primary Narcissism and Primary Love', *Psycho-Analytic Quarterly* 29(1): 6–43. Reprinted in *The Basic Fault: Therapeutic Aspects of Regression*, London: Tavistock Publications, 1968, pp. 34–76.

1960b 'Examination by the Patient', *Excerpta Medica* 53: 9–14. Reprinted in *Psychotherapeutic Techniques in Medicine* (with Enid Balint), London: Tavistock Publications, 1961, pp. 47–60.

1961 (with Enid Balint) *Psychotherapeutic Techniques in Medicine*, London: Tavistock Publications.

1962 'The Theory of Parent–Infant Relationship', *International Journal of Psycho-Analysis* 43(4–5): 251–2. Reprinted in *Primary Love and Psychoanalytic Technique* (2nd, rev. and enlarged edn), London: Tavistock Publications, 1965, pp. 145–7.

1963a 'The Younger Sister and Prince Charming', *International Journal of Psycho-Analysis* 44(2): 226–7.

1963b 'The Benign and the Malignant Forms of Regression', *Bulletin of the Association of Psycho–analytic Medicine* 3(2), pp. 20–8. Reprinted in *The Basic Fault: Therapeutic Aspects of Regression*, London: Tavistock Publications, 1968, pp. 117–56.

1964 *The Doctor, His Patient and the Illness* (2nd, rev. and enlarged edn), London: Pitman Medical.

1965 *Primary Love and Psychoanalytic Technique* (2nd, rev. and enlarged edn), London: Tavistock Publications.

1966a (with Enid Balint, R. Gosling and P. Hildebrand) *A Study of Doctors*, London: Tavistock Publications.

1966b 'Psychoanalysis and Medical Practice', *International Journal of Psycho-Analysis* 47(1): 54–62.

1968 *The Basic Fault: Therapeutic Aspects of Regression*, London: Tavistock Publications.

1969 'Trauma and Object Relationship', *International Journal of Psycho-Analysis* 50: 429–36.

1970a (with N. Hunt, D. Joyce, M. Mainker and J. Woodcock) *Treatment or Diagnosis: a Study of Repeat Prescriptions in General Practice*, London: Tavistock Publications.

1970b 'La Genèse de mes idées', *Gazette Médical, France* 77(3): 457–66.

1972 (with Enid Balint and P.H. Ornstein) *Focal Psychotherapy – an Example of Applied Psychoanalysis*, London: Tavistock Publications.

References

Balint, A. (1939) 'Love for the Mother and Mother Love', in M. Balint, *Primary Love and Psychoanalytic Technique*, London: Hogarth Press (1952).

Balint, E. and Norrel, J. (eds) (1973) *Six Minutes for the Patient*, London and New York: Tavistock Publications.

Balint, E., Courtenay, M., Elder, A., Hull, S. and Julian, P. (1993) *The Doctor, the Patient and the Group*, London and New York: Routledge.

Bion, W. (1962) 'A Theory of Thinking', *International Journal of Psycho-Analysis*, 43: 306–10.

—— (1963) *Elements of Psychoanalysis*, London: Heinemann.

Bollas, C. (1987) *The Shadow of the Object: Psychoanalysis of the Unthought Known*, London: Free Association Books.

Bowlby, J. (1969) *Attachment and Loss*, vol. 1, *Attachment*, London: Hogarth.

—— (1973) *Attachment and Loss*, vol. 2, *Separation*, London: Hogarth.

—— (1975) 'Attachment Theory, Separation Anxiety and Mourning', in D.A. Hamburg and H.K. Brodie (eds) *The American Handbook of Psychiatry*, vol. 6, New York: Basic Books.

—— (1980) *Attachment and Loss*, vol. 3, *Loss*, London: Hogarth.

Clyne, M. (1961) *Night Calls*, London: Tavistock Publications.

Clyne, M., Hawes, A.J., Lask, A. and Saville, P.R. (1963) 'The Discontented Patient', *Journal of the College of General Practitioners* 6: 87–102.

Courtenay, M. (1968) *Sexual Discord in Marriage*, London: Tavistock Publications.

Elder, A. and Samuel, O. (eds) (1987) *While I'm Here, Doctor*, London: Tavistock Publications.

Fairbairn, R. (1953) *Psychoanalytic Studies of the Personality*, London: Routledge.

—— (1963) 'Synopsis of an Object-relations Theory of the Personality', *International Journal of Psycho-Analysis* 44: 224–6.

Ferenczi, S. (1924) *Thalassa: a Theory of Genitality*, London: Karnac Books (1989).

—— (1932) 'Notes and Fragments', in *Final Contributions*, London: Hogarth.

—— (1933) 'Confusion of Tongues', in *Final Contributions*, London: Hogarth.

—— (1988) *Clinical Diary*, J. Dupon (ed.), Cambridge, MA: Harvard University Press.

Freud, S. (1914) 'Remembering, Repeating and Working-through', SE 12 (*Standard Edition of the Complete Psychological Works of Sigmund Freud*), London: Hogarth Press.

—— (1919) 'Lines of Advance in Psychoanalytic Therapy', SE 17.

—— (1937) 'Analysis Terminable and Interminable', SE 23.

Friedman, L. (1962) *Virgin Wives*, London: Tavistock Publications.

Gosling, R. (1978) 'Internalization of the Trainer's Behaviour in Professional Training', *British Journal of Medical Psychology* 51: 35–40.

Greenberg, J.R. and Mitchell, S.A. (1983) *Object Relations in Psychoanalytic Theory*, Cambridge, MA: Harvard University Press.

Haynal, A. (1988) *The Technique at Issue*, London: Karnac Books.

Hopkins, P. (1960) 'Psychiatry in General Practice', *Postgraduate Medical Journal* 36: 323–30.

Khan, M.M.R. (1969) 'On the Clinical Provision of Frustrations, Recognitions and Failures in the Analytic Situation', *International Journal of Psycho-Analysis* 50: 237–48.

—— (1972) 'Dread of Surrender to Resourceless Dependence in the Analytic Situation', *International Journal of Psycho-Analysis* 53: 225–30.

Lask, A. (1966) *Asthma, Attitude and Milieu*, London: Tavistock Publications.

Little, M. (1985) 'Winnicott Working in Areas where Psychotic Anxieties Predominate: a Personal Record', *Free Associations* 3: 9–42.

Malan, D. (1963) *A Study of Brief Psychotherapy*, London: Tavistock Publications.

Morse, S. (1972) 'Structure and Reconstruction: a Critical Comparison of Michael Balint and D.W. Winnicott', *International Journal of Psycho-Analysis* 53: 487–500.

Pedder, J. (1976) 'Attachment and New Beginning: Some Links between the Work of Michael Balint and John Bowlby', in G. Kohon (ed.) *The British School of Psychoanalysis: the Independent Tradition*, London: Free Association Books.

Rayner, E. (1991) *The Independent Mind in British Psychoanalysis*, London: Free Association Books.

Rickman, J. (1951) 'Number and the Human Sciences', in *Selected Contributions on Psychoanalysis*, London: Hogarth Press (1957).

Riviere, J. (1952) 'On the Genesis of Psychical Conflict in Earliest Infancy', in *Developments in Psychoanalysis*, London: Hogarth Press.

Spillius, E.B. (1983) 'Some Developments from the Work of Melanie Klein', *International Journal of Psycho-Analysis* 64: 321–32.

Stern, D. (1985) *The Interpersonal World of the Infant*, New York: Basic Books.

Stewart, H. (1989) 'Technique at the Basic Fault: Regression', *International Journal of Psycho-Analysis* 70: 221–30, and in *Psychic Experience and Problems of Technique*, London and New York: Routledge (1992).

—— (1992) 'Clinical Aspects of Malignant Regression', *Contemporary Psychotherapeutic Review* 7: 25–41 and in *The Legacy of Sandor Ferenczi*, L. Aron and A. Harris (eds), Hillsdale, NJ and London: Analytic Press (1993).

Sutherland, J.D. (1980) 'The British Object Relations Theorists: Balint, Winnicott, Fairbairn, Guntrip', *Journal of the American Psychoanalytic Association* 28: 829–60.

Winnicott, D.W. (1952) 'Psychoses and Child Care', in *Collected Papers: Through Paediatrics to Psychoanalysis*, London: Tavistock Publications (1958).

—— (1954) 'Metapsychological and Clinical Aspects of Regression within the Psychoanalytical Set-up', in *Collected Papers: Through Paediatrics to Psychoanalysis*, London: Tavistock Publications (1958).

—— (1963) 'The Development of the Capacity for Concern', in *The Maturational Processes and the Facilitating Environment*, London: Hogarth Press (1965).

—— (1969) 'The Use of an Object', *International Journal of Psycho-Analysis* 50: 711–16.

—— (1987) *The Spontaneous Gesture: Selected Letters*, F.R. Rodman (ed.) Cambridge, MA and London: Harvard University Press.

Name index

Preliminary note: Michael Balint's name is abbreviated to MB throughout

Abraham, Karl 16

Balint, Alice 1, 2, 3, 23, 25, 27
Balint, Enid 3
Balint, Enid 3, 4; applied work 12,
  84, 87, 90, 99, 110, 112, 113; and
  Family Discussion Bureau 86, 89;
  theoretical work 12, 45
Balint, John 3
Bergsmann (family) 1
Bergsmann, Emmi 1
Bergsmann, father of MB 1, 3
Bergsmann, mother of MB 3
Bion, W. 9, 50, 56, 78
Bollas, Christopher 76–7
Bowlby, John 25, 71, 72

Casement, Patrick 75
Clyne, M. 84, 99
Courtenay, M. 84, 87

Dormandi, Olga 3

Eichholz, Enid *see* Balint, Enid
Elder, Andrew 87, 99, 110

Fairbairn, W.R. 36–7, 44, 71, 72, 73,
  78; and hate 10, 19, 28
Fenichel, Otto 34
Ferenczi, Sandor 16, 36, 60, 88; and
  application of psychoanalysis to

medical practice 12, 83;
  'Confusion of Tongues between
  the Adults and the Child' 17, 48,
  49, 62; and hatred 28; MB's
  analysis with 2, 6; as model for
  MB 6; and object relations 8, 19,
  78; and parapsychology 35, 49;
  and 'passive object-love' 20; and
  regression 7, 53, 54, 56, 59, 73,
  74; 'super-ego introspression' 64;
  and training analysis 65; and
  transference–counter-transference
  relationship 23; and trauma 11, 17,
  62
Freud, A. 56
Freud, Sigmund 2, 9, 16, 19, 22, 78;
  and analytic work 17; and
  application of psychoanalysis to
  medical practice 83; classical
  technique 52; and hatred 10, 28;
  and libido 37; MB reads 1, 15; as
  model for MB 6; and narcissism
  50–1; and parapsychology 35, 49;
  and regression 7, 53–4, 56, 73; and
  training analysis 65; and trauma 61,
  62; and working-through 7, 18, 47
Friedman, L. 84

Gosling, Robert 84, 90, 96
Greenberg, Jay 72–4
Guntrip, H. 72

Subject index

development 20–1, 73
ego 26, 29, 70–1; early development
of 22–5, 51; and training 64
ego-psychology, psychoanalytic 63
ego skills of philobat 40
environment 7, 21, 24, 39
environment-mother (Winnicott) 21
'Eros and Aphrodite' 21–2
European Psychoanalytical
Federation, English-Speaking
Conferences 4
evocation (Bollas) 76
'Examination by the Patient' 103

fairy tales 42
false-self organization (Winnicott) 9
Family Discussion Bureau 4, 84, 86,
89
family planning 84
Family Planning Association 4, 12,
84, 86
Family Welfare Association 3
'Final Goal of Psychoanalytic
Treatment, The' 18
Focal Psychotherapy 12, 84, 86
focal therapy 4, 12, 85–6
free associations 29, 102
free-floating attention 102
Freudians 25; *see also* Freud *in Name
Index*
frustration 31, 37, 44; *see also*
gratification
fugues 42
fun-fairs 38, 39

general practice 111; changes in, and
MB's contribution 4, 11–12,
99–100; *see also* GPs
genital object-love 32
genital-orgastic elements in
transference 57
GP training 99–100; *see also* Balint
groups
GPs: consulting style 112; account of
their use of Balint groups 111–29;
effects of Balint groups on
professional competence 107–10;

gains from Balint groups 96–9,
101–2, 109; *see also* doctor–patient
relationship
gratification of wishes and desires in
analysis 23–4, 25, 28, 31, 33, 54,
55, 56, 57, 72, 73, 74, 77; *see also*
physical contact
group dynamics 95

hallucination 42
Hannah V: descriptive example 124–9
harmony: in object relationships 9,
27; primary object-love as
harmonious state 8, 11, 39, 41–2,
51, 55, 75–6
hate 9–10, 19, 27–9, 33, 70, 72; and
thrills 41; and training analysis 66
holding function of mother
(Winnicott) 56
homosexual patients 75: descriptive
example 114–18; focal therapy
with latent 86
homosexuality 15
human relationships 3; MB's interest
in development of 1, 15
Hungarian Psychoanalytical Society 2
Hungary: political situation 1–2
hysteria 26, 30, 57, 78

id 29, 73
idealization 44, 53; in training analysis
66, 67
idealized object 33, 66
illusion 42
impingement, theory of (Winnicott) 9
infancy: feeding rhythms in 3, 34; and
origins of basic fault 9, 49–50
infantile development 8–10, 22–6, 31,
39, 41, 42, 78–9; *see also* libido;
primary object-love
instincts, aggressive 39
instinctual drives 38–9, 73, 78
instinctual object-relations 8, 24, 78
Institute of Marital Studies 4, 84, 86, 89
Institute of Psychosexual Medicine 4,
12, 86
internal objects 72, 107